Style Rx

Bridgette Raes

Style Rx

Dressing the **Body You Have** to Create the **Body You Want**

Photography by
Lori Berkowitz

A Perigee Book

A PERIGEE BOOK
Published by the Penguin Group
Penguin Group (USA) Inc.
375 Hudson Street, New York, New York 10014, USA
Penguin Group (Canada), 90 Eglinton Avenue East, Suite 700, Toronto, Ontario M4P 2Y3, Canada
(a division of Pearson Penguin Canada Inc.)
Penguin Books Ltd., 80 Strand, London WC2R 0RL, England
Penguin Group Ireland, 25 St. Stephen's Green, Dublin 2, Ireland (a division of Penguin Books Ltd.)
Penguin Group (Australia), 250 Camberwell Road, Camberwell, Victoria 3124, Australia
(a division of Pearson Australia Group Pty. Ltd.)
Penguin Books India Pvt. Ltd., 11 Community Centre, Panchsheel Park, New Delhi—110 017, India
Penguin Group (NZ), 67 Apollo Drive, Rosedale, North Shore 0632, New Zealand
(a division of Pearson New Zealand Ltd.)
Penguin Books (South Africa) (Pty.) Ltd., 24 Sturdee Avenue, Rosebank, Johannesburg 2196, South Africa

Penguin Books Ltd., Registered Offices: 80 Strand, London WC2R 0RL, England

While the author has made every effort to provide accurate telephone numbers and Internet addresses at the time of publication, neither the publisher nor the author assumes any responsibility for errors, or for changes that occur after publication. Further, the publisher does not have any control over and does not assume any responsibility for author or third-party websites or their content.

First edition: January 2008

Library of Congress Cataloging-in-Publication Data

Raes, Bridgette.
    Style rx : dressing the body you have to create the body you want / Bridgette Raes ; photography by Lori Berkowitz
        p. cm.
    Includes index.
    ISBN 978-0-399-53387-7
    1. Clothing and dress. 2. Fashion. 3. Beauty, Personal. I. Title.
    TT507.R23 2008
    746.9'2—dc22   2007028068

PRINTED IN THE UNITED STATES OF AMERICA

10 9 8 7 6 5 4 3 2 1

This book is dedicated to my father,

John Raes

Contents

Contents

Introduction

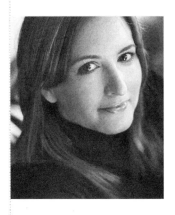

WHY ARE YOU picking up this book?

Maybe it's because you have finally accepted that when it comes to choosing the right clothing, you feel lost without a map. Maybe the idea of getting a bikini wax seems more appealing than shopping for pants. Or perhaps you're frustrated with the size of your thighs or tired of buying clothes that make you look worse rather than better. Whatever the reason, you've come to the right place.

With this book, I'm going to share with you all the answers that you need to choose the perfect clothes for your body, so that you can make better clothing decisions (that you will actually wear); stop the vicious cycle of a wardrobe full of unworn clothes (with tags still attached); and begin to feel great in what you wear, giving you greater confidence, a sense of mastery in an area where you often feel clueless, and an ease and enjoyment in actually finding the right clothing.

The advice and strategies in this book aren't just canned theories that *might* work. Each solution is based on real clients and what truly helped them master the art of dressing their bodies. I spent ten years working as a fashion designer, trained as an image consultant, and have spent the past five years running an image and style consulting company in New York City, teaching hundreds of women these tips and strategies. While I started this business with a background in fashion, the hands-on situations with clients are what have strengthened and perfected what I am going to share with you. I have seen every client in her underwear, have talked clients off the emotional ledge when they can't get the fifth pair of pants on while nudging them to try on one more pair. I have seen how one seam, button placement, or neckline can make a world of difference, and now I am taking these strategies out of the dressing room and sharing them with you.

Lost in the dressing room

Does this sound familiar? You're standing in the dressing room struggling to get a pair of pants over your thighs. You look at the size on the label and can't believe these pants don't fit. Frustrated, you think, *I have to get back to the gym.* After numerous trips to the sales racks, you finally discover pants that you may be able to get on, but now you can't believe how bad you look. You crane your neck around and look at yourself in the mirror from behind. *When did my butt get so big?* you wonder. *I have to stop eating after six p.m., or better yet, I have to stop eating, period.*

Whether it's a big butt, large thighs, a flat chest, a too-buxom chest, or some other problem area, we have all had these frustrating moments in the dressing room. We make purchases we're not satisfied with, ending up with clothes in our closet that we either don't wear or find uncomfortable or unflattering. We feel bad about the way we look, desperate to lose weight, guilty for making impractical purchases, and exhausted from trying.

Yet it doesn't have to be like this.

Clothing can be an amazing tool *if* it's chosen properly for a particular job. The right pair of pants can make you look five pounds lighter. That shirt with the perfect neckline can make you look leaner, taller, and more balanced. The dress that seems like it was made just for you can add a spring to your step. When you know what the right choices are for your particular body, suddenly the shame and frustration that you have about your image starts to dissipate.

It is my hope that by using this book, you'll find clothing that is right for your body—regardless of the shape of your thighs, the size of your chest, or the length of your legs. Instead of feeling depressed or suffering through a crash diet, plastic surgery, or other body-altering measures, you'll discover that it's never your body that's bad for the clothing, but that it's particular clothing that's a bad match for your body. You'll learn to seek out the cuts and shapes that will accentuate your positive features and make the best of your challenging ones. Rather than focusing on the size you wear, you'll be taught how to break down your body, part by part, and how to dress each part for the best look for you.

The body type dilemma

Many fashion and style experts try to help women solve their body issues by classifying their body type. If you have large thighs, then you're a pear. Have a tummy? You're an apple. These distinctions, while helpful for some women, do have flaws. You may have a pear shape because your hip size seems to match this category. But what about the large ankles that make it hard to fit into a pair of boots? Or the long torso that makes it impossible to keep your shirt tucked in? Additionally, some women don't seem to fit any type at all, leaving them completely powerless to make a smart decision.

The truth is that each woman's body is completely unique—a mixed bag of body components. The Style Rx approach embraces this diversity. Rather than asking you to focus on one overall body type—a type that might not address your individual concerns—I want you to take a part-by-part approach to dressing your best. Think of it as the fashion equivalent of a children's flip book, giving you the ability to customize your own dressing plan.

As you move through these pages, you'll notice that the principles I share for body challenges work for a spectrum of sizes. You may be a petite size 2 but have trouble fitting your butt into pants, or you may be a tall size 10 and have the same issue. The solution for both situations is the same.

The base body proportions we are born with stay with us no matter what size we are. If you collect weight in your thighs, whatever size you wear, your thighs will always be your area of concern. Body issues don't go away when we lose weight; they just get proportionately smaller. Getting hung up about the size on the label is useless; instead, it is smarter to focus on the proportions of your body and how to make the wisest clothing choices.

In addition, women go through changes. Giving birth and something as simple as gravity can cause certain body parts to droop south. Our hips, feet, and even our backs can widen after bearing children, adding more body concerns than the ones we are born with and that remain with us throughout our lives. So in addition to using this book to learn how to dress your own unique body, you'll also find strategies that may be of use as your body changes due to pregnancy or age.

A quick note on the models used in this book: None of the women featured are professional models. Twelve of the seventeen models are clients whom I have worked with one on one, others are friends, and one is actually my sister. Like you, all these women deal every day with real body issues. Before our work together, they had little to no idea what clothing choices were best for their bodies. They were all winging it just like you may be doing. Yet with the principles I'm going to share with you, they've not only learned to choose the right clothing for their body but also gained a sense of empowerment, control, and—most important—acceptance of the body they have. As they have learned, and as you will, too, from reading this book, it's much easier to accept and embrace a body issue when you know what to do with it.

Sure, any woman, including many of the women in this book (and me, too, for that matter), would certainly trade away their body issues in a heartbeat. Do I stare in the mirror and push my thighs in, wishing they were a bit slimmer? Of course I do. I have gone head on with a pair of boots that I can't zip over my large calves, I have cursed my narrow shoulders for making my thighs look even wider, and I have found myself blaming the gene pool from which my body was created. So be assured, I am certainly not expecting any of you to read this book and throw a party celebrating your chunky arms. But what I am hoping is that you use this book to build a more empowered and positive relationship with your body by making informed and powerful clothing decisions that work specifically for you.

A one-size-fits-all solution: how to use this book

In Part I, we'll focus on the problem areas that you know you have—those nagging spots that you would be happy to trade in or get rid of forever if you had the chance. Using the Style Rx CASE method, we'll find ways to dress around these challenges. There may be a few or many issues with which you identify. By going through them part by part, you'll self-diagnose the different components that make up your body, go to the relevant sections to create a personalized body plan, and then move to Part II for the next steps.

You will notice there are several strategies for each body issue. While it is important to address each concern separately, you also have to look at your body as a whole. Some of the advice given for a specific body concern may contradict a strategy for another body issue that you have. Therefore, the approach is to break your body down piece by piece and then choose the specific strategies that support your whole body.

In Part II, we'll discuss the most important part of the dressing equation: you. While it's important to choose the right clothing for your body issues, all these strategies can quickly become a wash if particular attention isn't paid to you shining in the end. The most important question we'll ask in Part II is:

> Are you wearing your clothing,
> or is your clothing wearing you?

In Part III, we will pull it all together with case studies of our models from this book using the CASE method. We'll look at each woman, learn about her body challenges, and then see the CASE method in action as we work toward a balanced look. This part will fully illustrate how each body issue affects the others, and how, in order to achieve complete body balance, you must diagnose each problem individually as well as looking at your body in its entirety.

I want you to feel empowered when you finish

this book, with a fresh perspective of your body. Each woman pictured in this book is built differently, and as I have always said, if there was supposed to be one standard body type for a woman that is considered perfect, then all of us would have been built the same. Instead of shaming our diversity, let's embrace it and redefine perfection, starting here with the Style Rx.

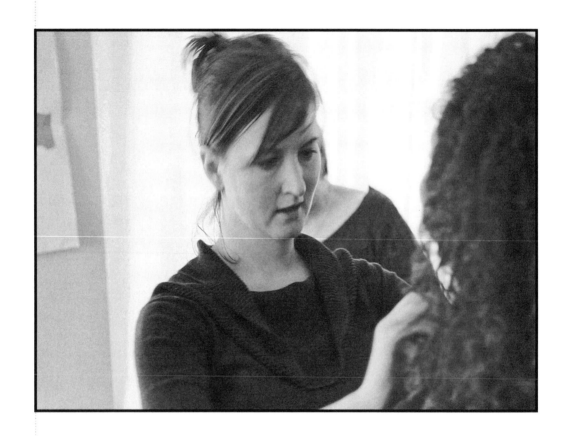

PART I

Diagnosis and Prescription

IN THIS PART, you will learn to identify and diagnose your specific body challenges and learn how to choose the right clothing to address each issue. In addition, you'll find out *why* each strategy works. Be ready for some "aha!" moments in which you finally solve those dressing problems you always recognized but never knew what to do about.

I certainly could have just given you the rules without much explanation or photography to back them up, but I felt it was important not only to give you the solution but also to explain in detail why each suggestion works. The more information you have, the more success you can have in the future. I also wanted to present these strategies in the simplest and most approachable manner possible, and that solution is what I call the CASE method.

Your Body and the CASE Method

THE CASE METHOD is a four-part strategy designed to help you work around your body challenges, enhance your assets, and develop the best look possible for your unique body. With the CASE method, you'll learn to create your own customized style solution—a "prescription" for your unique shape, one that will help you feel confident about the clothing you wear and the body you wear it on!

The CASE method is not about hiding or ignoring the challenges you may encounter. What it is about is balance and learning how to develop a better relationship with your body.

Because so many of us have chosen to fight the body challenges we have been given, through crash dieting and squeezing into clothing that we wished flattered us but doesn't, few of us have learned to make the best of what we have. Frustration arises not only from having the issue but also from having no idea how to solve it.

In my years of private consulting with women, I have never met two with the same exact body characteristics. Yet even though we are all built differently, many of us are striving to fit into the same singular mold of perceived perfection. When we apply the CASE method to dressing ourselves, not only do we embrace our diversity but we develop a more powerful relationship with our appearance, using clothing as a tool to enhance our assets and make us feel more beautiful and confident.

The CASE method is composed of the following components/strategies:

Counterbalance
Angle
Shape and/or **S**horten
Elongate

Let's explore what each one of these strategies means.

▶ **Counterbalance.** Counterbalance means to add width or weight to one body area, such as the shoulders, to compensate for the natural width or fullness of an opposite area, such as the hips—the result is an illusion of balance.

▶ **Angle.** Angles are diagonal lines or diagonal shapes created in the silhouette of clothing. Wherever you add angles in your wardrobe, you create a slimming and minimizing line to that area.

▶ **Shape.** To shape literally means to add shape to a body characteristic. While shaping seems like an obvious strategy, it is one of the most overlooked yet most effective ways of dressing in a balanced manner. When a woman isn't happy with a particular body characteristic, she tends to shy away from shaping that area and instead hides out in shapeless unflattering clothing. Yet by shaping an area, you can actually look slimmer.

▶ **Shorten.** Like shaping, the meaning of shortening is pretty obvious. In addition to decreasing the length of an area that is longer, shortening can also be used to widen or create fullness in slimmer areas.

▶ **Elongate.** When you elongate an area of your body, you not only create length but also narrow and slim that area.

Now that you know what the CASE method consists of, it's time to start using these strategies to find the power and knowledge you need to love the way you look.

The Total Body Checklist

IN THIS PART, you'll identify all the physical challenges you'll want to address through the CASE method and learn how to select clothing that compensates for these issues. You may also have body areas or features that you consider average or not an issue. Since this book isn't about creating more problems for you to face, feel free to skip any sections that don't relate to your concerns.

To begin, I recommend reading this book with a notebook in hand, in which you can take your own notes and record your own overall body strategy. You may want to add some personal thoughts and ideas while reading and strategizing. I also recommend having some recent photographs of your face and full body that you can refer to while reading, as it will be a lot easier to study pictures instead of running back and forth to the mirror each time you want to self-diagnose.

I also suggest sharing this book with your friends. By sharing your findings about your body with your friends, who can also share their findings with you, you'll find that each body characteristic addressed in this book has its share of pluses and minuses. We all spend so much time wishing our bodies were different or thinking that our friends who have bodies opposite ours can't have the problems that we do. After writing this book and exploring each body characteristic in detail, I can confidently say that there isn't one body characteristic that has it any easier than any other. In addition, it will be interesting to see just how much diversity you and your friends share.

Your neck:
- If you have a short neck, go to page 8.
- If you have a long neck, go to page 14.

You may not be sure if you have a short neck or not. Here is a quick test: Without strain or effort, drop your chin to your chest. If your chin rests easily or comes close to resting on your chest, then your neck is short. If your neck comes nowhere near touching your chest, then your neck is long.

Your shoulders:
- If you have narrow shoulders, go to page 20.
- If you have broad shoulders, go to page 26.

Your chest:
- If you have a small chest, go to page 32.
- If you have a large chest, go to page 38.

Your arms:
- If you have large arms, go to page 44.
- If you have thin arms, go to page 50.
- If you have long arms, go to page 56.

Do you have long arms? Standing in front of a mirror with your arms at your sides, look at where your thumbs hit your body. If your arms are longer than your crotch, then you have long arms.

Your waist:
- If you have a short waist, go to page 62.
- If you have a long waist, go to page 68.

Do you have a short waist or a long waist? If you aren't sure if your waist is short or long, take two measurements. First, measure the distance from your armpit to your natural waist. (Your natural waist is found right around the area of your belly button and where you rest your hands at your waist.) Second, measure from your natural waist to where your crotch point is. Your crotch point is the point on your body where the pelvis ends and the legs begin. If the measurement from your armpit to your waist is shorter than the measurement from your waist to your crotch, then you have short waist. If the measurement from your armpit to your waist is longer than the measurement from your waist to your crotch point, then you have a long waist.

- If you have a slight waist, go to page 74.
- If you have a tummy, go to page 80.

Your hips:

> ▶ If you have wide hips, go to page 86.
>
> ▶ If you have narrow hips, go to page 92.

Your butt:

> ▶ If you have a big butt, go to page 98.
>
> ▶ If you have a flat butt, go to page 104.

Your thighs:

> ▶ If you have large thighs, go to page 110.

Your legs:

> ▶ If you have short legs, go to page 116.
>
> ▶ If you have long legs, go to page 122.

Your calves and ankles:

> ▶ If you have large calves and ankles, go to page 128.
>
> ▶ If you have thin calves and ankles, go to page 134.

Your feet:

> ▶ If you have wide feet, go to page 140.
>
> ▶ If you have narrow feet, go to page 146.

Short Neck

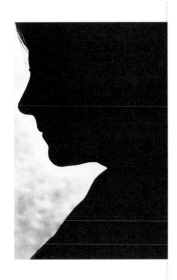

IF YOU HAVE a short neck, you probably find yourself admiring women with long, swanlike necks, frustrated because you wonder how you, too, can have this same languid grace without hanging yourself by your ears, doing crazy neck exercises, or stretching your neck with rings.

Even if you are tall, your neck may make you feel short, squat on top, and as if you are constantly hunching. Dressing options, in particular with necklines, seem more limited. Turtlenecks make you feel like a turtle, chokers may actually choke you, and dangly chandelier earrings literally graze your shoulders.

To look more physically balanced, you don't have to walk around imagining that a string is pulling your head toward the sky or stretching your neck like a giraffe. After all, you aren't looking to graze the treetops for a savory leaf—you just want your neck to look longer. With the CASE method strategies, I am going to show you how to make that happen.

The best way to make something that is short look longer is to elongate it—the perfect element of the CASE method for those of you with shorter necks.

elongate

- ▶ Shorter earrings visually create the look of a longer neck by creating more visual space between your ears and your shoulders, therefore making your neck look longer.
- ▶ The more space you create around your neck through deeper necklines, the longer your neck will appear. Turtlenecks have the opposite effect and make your neck look shorter.
- ▶ Longer necklaces and scarves that hang long around your neck lengthen the look of your neck.
- ▶ Horizontal lines placed anywhere on the body have a shortening effect; therefore, horizontal necklines such as boatnecks shorten the look of your neck. Choose deeper necklines or necklaces that don't cut across the base of your neck in such a horizontal manner.

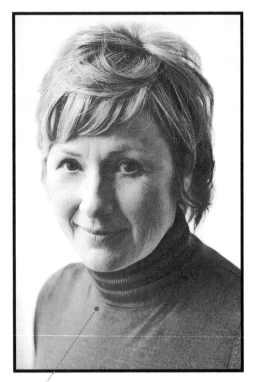

The neck is shortened with a turtleneck.

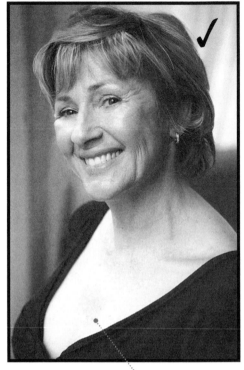

The neck is elongated with a deeper neckline.

The more you open up the space around your neck, the longer it will appear. In the photo on the left, the fabric of the turtleneck travels right up to our model's chin, making her neck appear shorter than it already is. Because our model is wearing a deeper and more open neckline in the photo on the right, her neck appears longer.

This does not mean that if you have a short neck you should swear off turtlenecks—after all, it does get cold! In situations where you want to wear a turtleneck, consider wearing a long necklace with your turtleneck or a more open cowl neck. A scarf hanging long around your neck will also have the same elongating effect because of the vertical lines it creates.

You can see that the longer earrings in the photo on the left are grazing our model's shoulders. Longer earrings have the potential of making your neck look shorter, especially when it looks as if you don't even have enough room between your ears and shoulders for them to hang freely.

If you look at the photo on the right, you'll see that our model's neck looks longer than it does in the photo on the left. The shorter earrings that she is wearing in the picture on the right create more visual space between her ears and her shoulders, therefore making her neck look longer.

Longer earrings are not to be avoided completely, but stay away from big, clunky attention grabbers and instead choose finer, more delicate ones. Avoid too much dangle or size. Anything larger than your eye socket can attract attention away from your face and make it hard for others to notice you over your earrings.

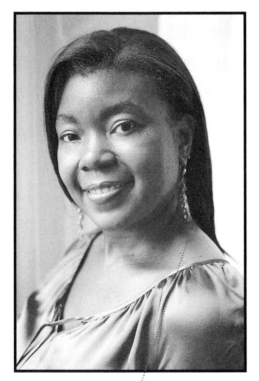

The neck is shortened with longer earrings.

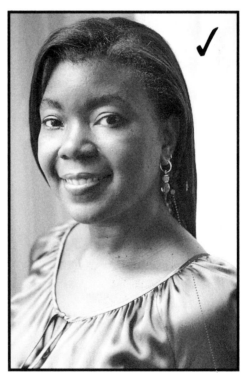

The neck is elongated with shorter earrings.

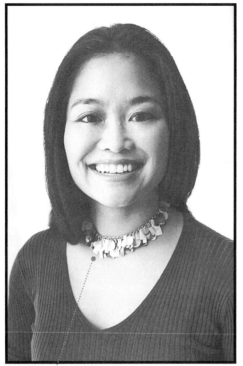

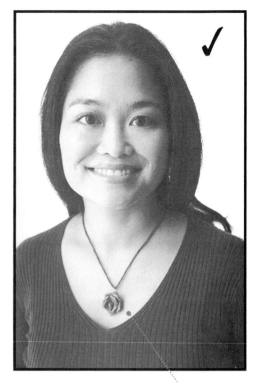

The neck is shortened with a choker.

The neck is elongated with a longer necklace.

When you have a short neck, the last thing you want to do is cut off the neck length you do have with a choker or a short necklace. In the photo on the left, the choker cuts off our model's neck and makes it appear shorter. In the photo on the right, she is wearing a longer necklace, and because of this, more space is opened up around her shorter neck, making it appear longer.

If you do have a longer neck and are going to choose a choker-style necklace, then choose the thinnest and finest style you can find. The chunkier it is, the shorter and squatter your neck will appear.

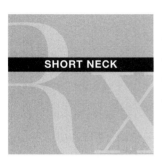

SHORT NECK

- Choose shorter earrings over longer ones.
- Avoid turtlenecks.
- Choose longer necklaces over chokers.
- Choose deeper necklines.

If you have a short neck . . .

▨ If a pair of long earrings graze your shoulders, take the earrings to a local jewelry repair shop and see if you can have them shortened.

▨ Try not to be so "buttoned up." If you have a short neck, unbutton your shirt as low as you feel comfortable. By opening up the space around your neck, it will appear longer. Another suggestion is to wear a tank top or camisole underneath your button-down shirts, giving you the ability to unbutton even lower while still covering up.

▨ A necklace with a strong pendant makes the neck appear longer. Avoid very beaded, clunky necklaces and instead choose thinner chains or chords with a more definite pendant.

quick tips

Long Neck

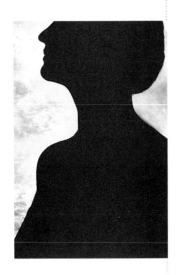

IF YOU HAVE a long neck, you know you're in good company: ballerinas, Audrey Hepburn, and swans—not so shabby! There is a languid gracefulness to a long neck that gives the appearance that you float with ease, rather than walk, throughout your day.

Sure, turtlenecks were made especially for a neck like yours, but there are times when you notice that your longer neck seems too long. There are also days when you don't want to look like you were born with a few extra vertebrae. Sometimes having a long neck makes you feel gangly or gawky, and slouching to make it appear shorter, which has seemed like your only solution, is starting to become a literal pain in the neck.

There is a way to look as if your head isn't literally in the clouds. With the strategies in this section, you're going to learn to balance your long swanlike neck without sacrificing the natural grace and elegance that comes with it.

The CASE strategy for balancing a long neck is to visually shorten it.

shorten

▶ Wherever you place a horizontal line, you shorten the area. Therefore, tying a scarf around your neck or wearing a choker-style necklace shortens the visual length of the neck by creating horizontal lines.

▶ A horizontal neckline, such as a boatneck, also makes your neck appear shorter. A deeper neckline, like that found in a deep V-neck, will have the opposite effect and make your neck appear longer.

▶ Necklaces that sit closer to the base of your neck have a shortening effect. Longer necklaces draw the eye downward, making your neck look even longer.

▶ Shirts with necklines that sit higher on the neck, like turtlenecks or collared shirts, also make your neck look shorter.

▶ Longer earrings make your neck look shorter because there is less space created between your earrings and your shoulders, and therefore the neck is shortened.

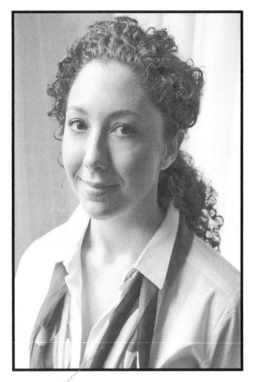

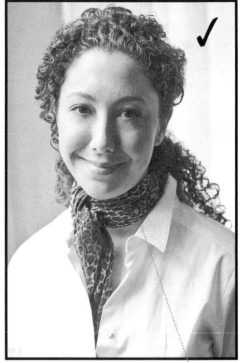

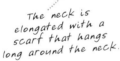
The neck is elongated with a scarf that hangs long around the neck.

The neck is shortened with a scarf that is tied around the neck.

Vertical lines elongate any area, so hanging a scarf long from the base of the neck adds unnecessary vertical length and makes the neck appear even longer. In the picture on the left, you can see the lengthening effects of the vertical lines. With a longer neck, the closer you wear your scarves and necklaces to your face, the shorter your neck will appear.

In the photo on the right, the model's neck is wrapped with a scarf, like a choker, making the neck appear shorter. Tying the scarf this way also connects her face more to the rest of her body by creating a visual connection between her head and her shoulders. Sometimes with a long neck, your face can appear disconnected from the rest of your body because the neck is so long, but by adding an element like a scarf to your neck area, your face and body become more synergized and connected.

Horizontal lines placed anywhere on the body shorten that area. By placing a horizontal line at the base of the neck, the appearance of a shorter neck is created.

The lower your neckline, the longer your neck will look. You can see in the photo on the left that the depth of the neckline makes the neck look longer. By wearing a higher neckline that sits closer to the base of your neck, or wearing a top like a turtleneck, the neck also looks shorter. You can see in the photograph on the right that our model's neck looks much shorter because of the higher neckline she is wearing.

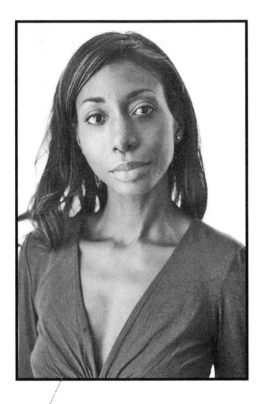

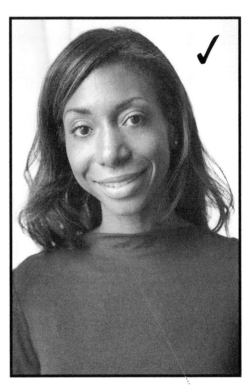

A long neck is elongated with a lower neckline.

A long neck is shortened with a higher neckline.

Diagnosis and Prescription

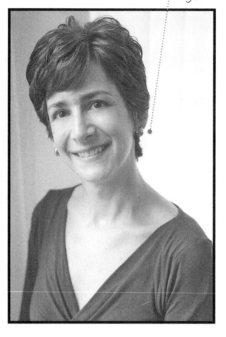

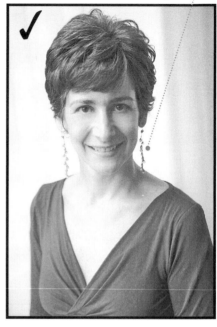

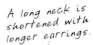

The best way to make your neck look more balanced and not so long is to wear longer earrings; by wearing longer earrings, there's less space between your ears and your neck, and your neck looks shorter.

To find the right length of earring, keep in mind the following rule of thumb: Your earrings should hang no longer than where your jawbone angles. To find this point, run your finger down your jawbone starting right below your earlobe until it starts to make a dramatic curve—that should be your maximum earring length.

Of course, as in the case of our model, there are many earring choices that extend much longer. This isn't wrong; however, when an earring hangs longer than where your jawline starts to angle, it detracts from your face and your earrings may stand out and overpower you. If you choose to wear these longer earrings, keep the rest of your outfit subtle to create more focus on the earrings. Additionally, longer earrings that hang past the point where your jawbone angles are okay if you don't need to hold someone's attention. If you do want someone to focus on you, as in an interview or a presentation, make sure your earrings are no longer than that angling point of your jawbone.

As you can see in the photo on the left, shorter earrings will make the neck look longer. If you want to wear shorter earrings, look for larger, more substantial ones or earrings that have a short drop and hang just below the ear.

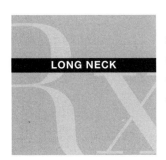

LONG NECK

- Tie scarves in a choker fashion.
- Wear higher necklines instead of deeper ones.
- Choose shorter necklaces instead of longer ones.
- Choose longer earrings over shorter ones.

If you have a long neck . . .

■ Long necks are usually very thin. To avoid making your long neck look too scrawny, don't wear cowl necks or wide turtlenecks that create a lot of space around your neck and make your neck look thinner. Choose turtle-neck styles that sit close to your neck.

■ Popping the collar, which means to slightly lift the back of a collar of a button-down shirt, frames your face and balances your neckline, yet doesn't cut off the gracefulness of your neck.

quick tips

Narrow Shoulders

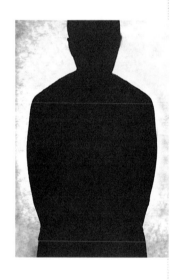

THERE IS A fine delicateness to a woman with narrow shoulders. Many artists, during the Renaissance period in particular, depicted these narrow-shouldered women as the ultimate beauty: sweet, feminine, and womanly. However, this isn't the Renaissance, and your narrow shoulders are not a feature you think should be depicted in art.

Because of the narrowness of your shoulder area, you have sometimes wondered if reverting back to the 1980s shoulder pad isn't such a bad idea, even if you run the risk of looking like a *Dynasty* reject. You may fight to keep your handbag from constantly slipping off your shoulder and often find yourself frustrated by bra straps that don't stay put. Additionally, because broad shoulders often exude a natural power and strength, you may feel that you look less strong than your broader-shouldered friends.

Narrow shoulders, while not usually considered the most challenging body issue by many, can have a negative impact on other body issues that you might consider to be a *very big* challenge. For example, narrow shoulders can emphasize a wider bottom half and make you feel that you look bottom heavy. Narrow shoulders are an example of how one body feature can strongly affect the appearance of other features if the right clothing choices aren't made.

While you can try to build your shoulders up with tons of exercise, and by being mindful of tossing your shoulders proudly back, your narrow shoulders are one of the body features that you can either get upset about or, instead, gain control of with the right clothing. In applying the CASE method for narrow shoulders, you will not only learn how to widen and broaden your shoulder area through clothing but also discover how doing this greatly impacts the appearance of the lower half of your body.

The CASE strategies for narrow shoulders are Counterbalance and Angle.

counterbalance

▶ A fuller skirt or pants make narrow shoulders look even narrower because the fullness at the bottom half of the body creates a narrower shoulder line. Instead, try a skirt that doesn't have too much fullness or straighter pants that sit closer to the legs.

angle

▶ Diagonal lines, such as stripes and ribbed stitching on a sweater, that angle toward the outer part of your shoulders make your shoulders look wider.

▶ Wider necklines such as boatnecks widen narrower shoulders because the width of the shoulder line makes the shoulders appear wider than they really are.

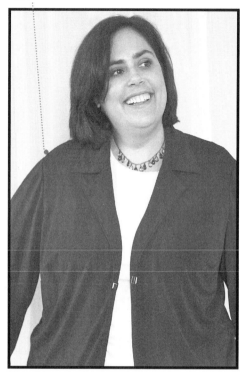

shoulders look narrower with a softer drop shoulder.

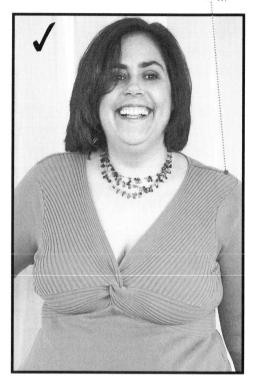

Shoulders look wider with lines that angle outward.

In the photo on the left, our model is wearing an unstructured jacket with a dropped shoulder. In dropped shoulder tops and jackets, the shoulder seam sits slightly off the shoulder and on the top half of the arm. This is never a good choice for anyone with narrow shoulders because this style creates a much softer shoulder line. As a result, the model's shoulders look narrower and more sloped than they already are. A raglan sleeve has the same shoulder-narrowing effect

as a dropped shoulder and should be avoided as well.

In the photo on the right, you can see how much wider our model's shoulders look because the ribbed knit at the neckline angles outward toward the wider part of the shoulder. Because these angled lines move in this direction, you see a wider shoulder. Stripes and seams that angle outward in this fashion have the same effect.

This model's shoulders are not as sloped as the ones we just looked at; however, her frame is so narrow that her shoulders, while squarer in shape, have an overall narrowness to them.

In the photo on the left, our model is wearing pants with full legs. Because her pants are wide, her shoulders appear narrow in relation to the width of the pants. As a result, her overall body shape looks more triangular rather than balanced between the top half and the lower half of her body. The same narrowing of the shoulders would happen if she wore a full skirt (versus a narrow skirt).

In the photo on the right, you can see that slimmer pants make her shoulders look broader and wider. This is because the slimness found in the lower half of her body makes the top half of her body appear wider.

The best way the model could balance her look with the pants she's wearing on the left is to pair them with a top that has a wider neckline or stripes that angle outward. Doing this would help make her shoulders look as wide as the bottom half of her body.

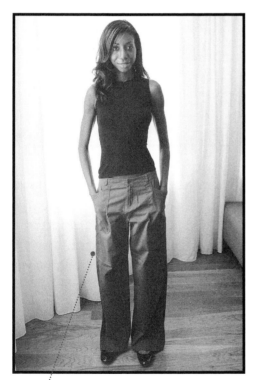

Shoulders are narrowed with wider pants.

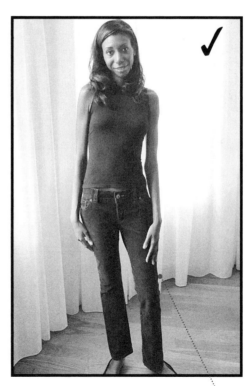

Shoulders are widened with narrower pants.

Diagnosis and Prescription

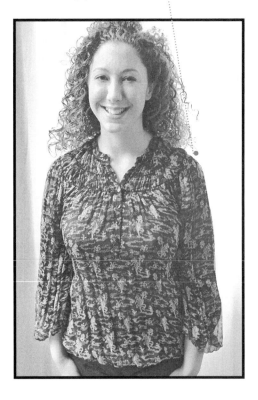

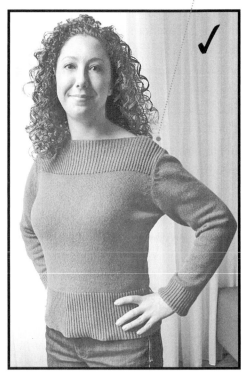

In the photo on the left, you can see that a softer shoulder line not only gives our model's shoulders a narrower and softer appearance but moves your focus toward the middle part of her body and away from her shoulder line. As a result, our model doesn't look as tall and thin. This is why many women with broad shoulders give off a strong, tall presence naturally. Women with narrower shoulders don't have as much of a natural ability to do this, which is why clothing that broadens the shoulders is so important.

In the picture on the right, a wider neckline broadens our model's narrow shoulders, because anywhere you place a horizontal line on the body, that area looks wider. What is also helping is the horizontal seam in the sweater that runs parallel to the horizontal neckline. Broadening narrow shoulders isn't just important for overall body balance; a stronger shoulder line also helps you appear taller because when the shoulders are broadened, the eye is directed upward.

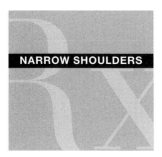

NARROW SHOULDERS

- Choose narrower bottoms over fuller bottoms.
- Choose diagonal lines that angle outward at the shoulder.
- Choose wider, square, or horizontally shaped necklines.

quick tips

If you have narrow shoulders . . .

■ Don't try to fool the eye with massive shoulders pads. If you wear large shoulder pads, it just looks like your shoulders are so narrow that you need the equivalent of football equipment to fill them out. Keep the bad 1980s shoulder pads out of your closet, and use a softer yet widening approach to broadening your shoulders, such as the tips shared here.

■ Choose armholes that sit properly on your shoulders. Shirts with armholes that are too narrow, like sleeveless tops that cut in too severely or halter tops, will make your shoulders look even narrower. Shirts with armholes that sit off your shoulders, like raglan sleeves, and shirts with drop armholes soften your shoulders and make them look more rounded.

■ Building up the shoulder with elements such as scarves and epaulets creates height and can make your shoulders appear wider.

Broad Shoulders

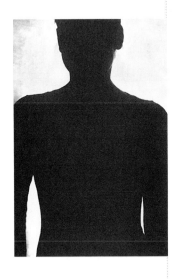

ANY WOMAN WITH broad shoulders will admit that there certainly are benefits that come with having a broad, square shoulder line. Your shoulders can give you a strong, powerful, and independent presence; clothing can drape from your body as if it were still on the hanger; and when exposed, a beautifully angled shoulder can be a striking sight.

Along with the advantages, however, you have your own share of challenges that leave you wishing you were as crafty as Michelangelo with a chisel. Yes, your shoulders look strong and powerful, but they sure can be bossy when it comes to dictating your clothing choices. Fitting your broad shoulders into a fine, delicate top or narrow jacket is as challenging as trying to get your cat into a carrier for its vet appointment—it is usually only with effort that you can be successful. You're probably familiar with the binding sensation that comes with having shoulders wider than what your shirt can contain, leaving you with only two choices: going one size up to fit your shoulders or buying clothing that fits at your waist but is too small for your shoulders, potentially ripping your shoulders right out of the seams. And shoulder pads? You certainly don't need them.

With the CASE strategies in this section, you'll learn how to make clothing decisions that will keep you from feeling like a permanent slouch is your only option for camouflaging your shoulders. You'll discover how to dress, knowing that your shoulders are a beautiful asset, rather than dressing and feeling like you're suiting up for a football game.

The four CASE strategies are effective for broad shoulders: Counterbalance, Angle, Shape, and Elongate.

counterbalance

▶ Full skirts or pants add width in opposition to your wider shoulders and counterbalance a broad shoulder line.

angle

▶ Angled lines that move inward toward your neck taper and slim your shoulders. Therefore, halter tops, V-necks, or any shirt with an angled neckline create a slimming effect and narrow the appearance of your shoulder line. Horizontal lines placed on any area of the body create added width. Avoid square necklines, boatnecks, or any neckline that cuts horizontally across your shoulder line; these necklines will only make your shoulders look wider.

shape

▶ Shirts with softer shoulder lines, such as those with softer armholes, raglan sleeves, or jackets or tops with either very small shoulder pads or no shoulder pads at all, are a good choice. You have your own personal shoulder pads; there's no need to add them!

elongate

▶ Vertical lines elongate an area and also make that area appear narrower and slimmer. Horizontal lines widen an area, so choose vertically striped tops over horizontal stripes.

▶ Longer necklaces and scarves that hang long around your neck create vertical lines and create a narrower shoulder line.

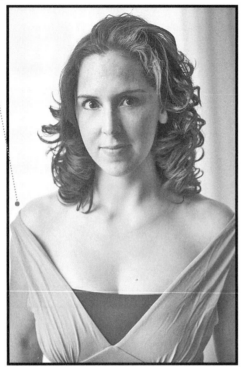

Broad shoulders are widened by angled lines that move outward toward the shoulder.

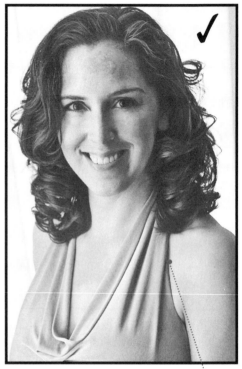

Broad shoulders are narrowed by angled lines that move inward.

In the picture on the left, a top that angles off our model's shoulders broadens her shoulder line because of the way the angled lines move outward. It forces your eye to see just how broad her shoulders are. Now you may be wondering, don't angled lines narrow an area? Even though the neckline of the top does angle, the wide angling directs your eye outward and creates the look of an even broader shoulder.

Additionally, the horizontal portion of her neckline in this photo mirrors the broad squareness of her shoulders, and by mirroring the square shape, her shoulders look even broader.

You can see in the picture on the right that the angle of the halter top softens the model's shoulder line because of the way the angle moves toward her neck. This movement forces your eye to move inward and therefore makes her shoulders appear narrower. The deep V-neck of the top also narrows her shoulders.

When choosing angles for your broad shoulders, it is important that the angles sit as close to your neck as possible.

The best way to minimize an area that is full or wide is to oppose it with fullness, or counterbalance.

In the photo on the right, you can see how the fullness of the skirt opposes her wide shoulders, creating a counterbalancing effect and making her shoulders look much narrower. You will notice that the top she is wearing tapers her shoulders because the armholes cut inward. The angle of the V-neck also creates the look of a narrower shoulder line because angles have a slimming effect.

In the photo on the left, you can see what happens when a more tapered skirt is worn by someone with broad shoulders. Because of the narrowness of the skirt, the broadness of her shoulders is emphasized. Instead of looking more balanced, she looks more top heavy or like an upside-down triangle.

This does not mean that if you have broad shoulders you can never wear a tapered or pegged skirt. What it does mean is that you must be wise about your top choices when you wear a narrow skirt. Had our model put on a top with a V-neckline or armholes that angled inward, her shoulders would be narrowed and the tapered skirt would look more balanced on her.

Broad shoulders are angled by a V-neckline.

Broad shoulders are narrowed with armholes that angle inward.

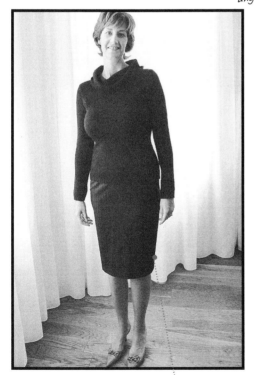

Broad shoulders are widened with a narrower skirt.

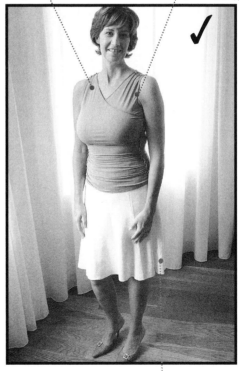

Broad shoulders are narrowed with a fuller skirt.

Diagnosis and Prescription

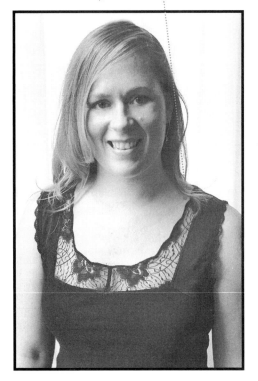

Shoulders are widened with a square neckline.

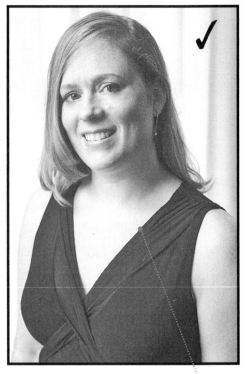

Shoulders are narrowed with an angled neckline.

These two pictures clearly show what a difference a neckline can make. Both of these tops are of the basic black sleeveless variety, something we all have in our wardrobe. The big difference is how each neckline affects broad shoulders.

In the photo on the left, you can see again what happens when you mirror a square shoulder with a horizontal line. Mirrors reflect, and by mirroring something that already exists, such as the squareness of our model's shoulders, you are just reflecting or emphasizing that thing.

In the picture on the right, you can see that the angled neckline softens and narrows her broad shoulders because angled lines narrow and minimize an area that is wide.

One of the best ways to balance an area is to do the opposite: instead of mirroring the shape that you want to minimize, go with an opposite shape.

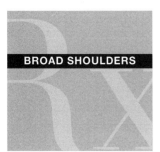

BROAD SHOULDERS

- Choose fuller bottoms over narrower ones.
- Choose diagonal lines that angle inward at the neck.
- Soften the shoulders with softer armholes.
- Choose vertical lines over horizontal lines.
- Choose V-necks over square necklines.

If you have broad shoulders . . .

▨ Broad shoulders can easily stretch out the shoulder area of a sweater. When possible, buy sweaters that have a high Lycra or spandex content, which will give your sweaters better recovery and the ability to bounce back into shape after you have worn them.

▨ Avoid ribbed knits, especially if they don't contain Lycra or spandex. While ribbed knits can shape your body well, ribbed sweaters have a tendency to stretch out easily and lose their ability to recover or bounce back after many wearings.

▨ To compensate for the width of your shoulders, you may find yourself buying shirts that are too big for the rest of your body, particularly your waist. A tailor can easily take your shirts in at the waist area and add darts to make them more shaped.

▨ Never buy shapeless tops without a defined waist shape; they will make you look like a big box. When considering the purchase of a knit top, lay it on a flat surface and make sure that there is waist definition or visible waist shaping.

quick tips

Diagnosis and Prescription

Small Chest

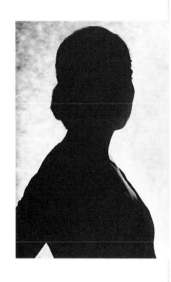

AS A YOUNG girl, you were probably told that when you hit puberty, your breasts would begin to develop. Embracing this possibility, you may have stared in the mirror with anxious anticipation for this rite of passage to start blossoming. But for you, an ample bustline never seemed to take form.

To make it look like this sign of womanhood didn't overlook you, you may have resorted to some not-so-savvy measures — stuffing tissues into your bras, applying gels and creams that promised to make your bust magically grow, and performing recommended exercises while repeating the mantra from the Judy Blume book: "We must, we must, we must increase our bust." As you matured and became a grown woman, you accepted that the boob fairy must have permanently misplaced your address, and those less sophisticated teenage measures led to more sophisticated solutions: buying bras with padding; purchasing silicone inserts; having a drawer full of bras all promising to increase cup size; and, for the really ambitious, getting surgical implants.

I can't blame you for wanting to magically create what isn't there. In our society, breasts are synonymous with womanhood. (How many beer ads and pinup calendars do we need to prove this point?) You may feel that you look boyish or masculine. Or you may feel ill-proportioned, not having enough curve on top to match the curve that you do have on the bottom.

Because clothing is oftentimes created for women with ample boobs, you may have a terrible time finding the right garments without bringing attention to what you don't have. But there are dressing options out there that work better for small-chested women than for women with larger chests. Additionally, there are clothing solutions that the smaller-chested gal can implement to create the look of a more ample bosom. So before you rush out and get plastic surgery, or drop another wad of cash on the bra that promises you will look like Mae West, let's take a look at the strategies designed specifically for you.

Shape and Elongate are the two effective CASE strategies that can help make a flat chest look fuller.

shape

▶ Choose a top with gathering in the bust area, which will enhance the fullness of your chest.

▶ Avoid shapeless jackets and tops that make you look like you can't fill out your clothes. Shaping in the waist creates the look of a larger chest.

elongate

▶ By wearing a higher neckline, you bring focus to your chest area and increase the illusion of shape. A deep V-neck brings attention to the fact that you can't fill out your top.

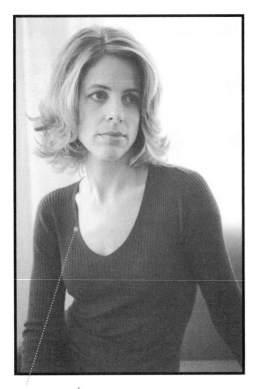

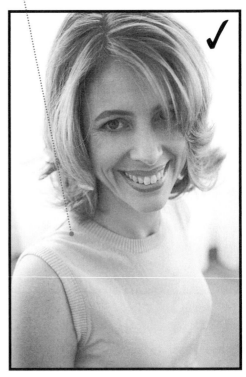

Small boobs look bigger with a higher neckline.

Small boobs look smaller with a plunging neckline.

Plunging necklines that show off your chest area, as in the photo on the left, also show off what is missing and the fact that she doesn't fill out her top. The deep V-neck also directs the eye downward, and the chest area doesn't look as full.

In the photo on the right, our model is wearing a shirt with a higher neckline, and you can see how much larger and fuller her chest looks. By elongating your chest area with a neckline that sits higher, the eye is directed upward and your bustline appears fuller, higher, and perkier.

In the photo on the left, you can see that a shapeless T-shirt just makes a small chest look smaller. Gathering creates shape and contour, something that smaller-chested women can use if they want to create a fuller and more ample bosom. The lack of gathering makes her chest look smaller.

The good news is that if you have a small chest, it doesn't mean that you need to swear off deep V-necks for the rest of your life. If you do want to wear a deeper neckline, I suggest that you choose a top with some gathering at the bust area, like the one our model is wearing in the photo on the right. The gathering creates fullness and helps add shape to the chest. This same principle applies to bathing suits as well. If you want to make your chest look larger, gathering in the bustline will make your chest look fuller versus a bandeau style, which will just flatten you.

Small boobs look smaller without gathering.

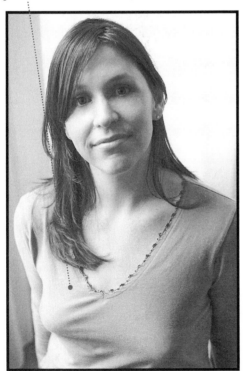

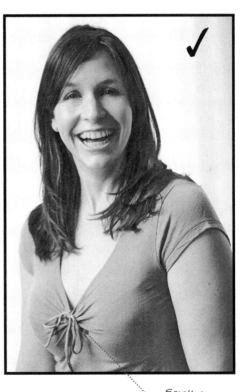

Small boobs look bigger with gathering.

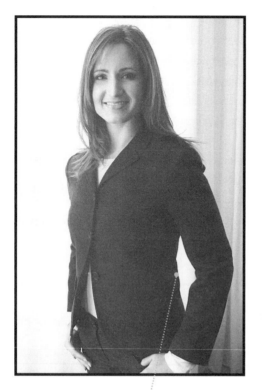

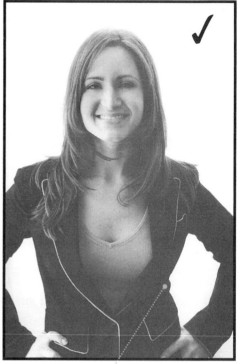

*Small boobs look
smaller in shapeless
jackets.*

*Small boobs
look bigger in
shaped jackets.*

In the photo on the left, you can see that the flat shapelessness of this jacket just makes our model's chest look smaller. The higher closing of this jacket also emphasizes how square and flat the jacket is and how it makes her look flat and square as a result.

In the photo on the right, you can see that the jacket has a lot of shape, and as a result, the model's bustline looks more shaped and fuller.

There is plenty of shape in the side seams and a lot of shaping created by the seaming found throughout the jacket. When buying a jacket, always choose one that emphasizes and shows off your waist area. The more shaped the top or jacket is, the more buxom you will appear. Additionally, the lower button closure of this jacket allows her bustline to show, which makes her chest look fuller.

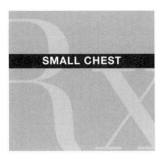

SMALL CHEST

- Add gathers at your bustline.
- Choose jackets with shape.
- Choose higher necklines over deeper necklines.

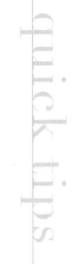

If you have a small chest . . .

- Avoid full shapeless tops and instead wear tops with shape, which give you a curvier and more buxom appearance.

- Add fullness by wearing ruffles, patch or flap pockets, or anything else eye-catching over your chest, and choose thicker cable-knit sweaters.

- Take advantage of the spaghetti straps and strapless clothing out there, which your larger-busted friends tend to avoid.

quick tips

Large Chest

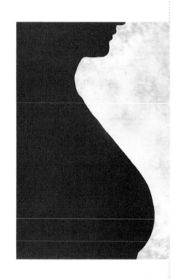

HAVING A LARGE chest can be both a blessing and a curse. Unlike your smaller-chested friends, who can get a padded bra or some other medieval contraption to "hike the girls up," being more ample in the bust department may make you feel as if you have far fewer options. You can't leave your boobs at home when you want to be perceived in a less sexual manner, you can't store them away in a gym locker when you want to do a power run on the treadmill, and you certainly have limited options when it comes to wearing something with spaghetti straps or, worse, no straps at all.

On the flip side, having a large chest is something that, when the time and situation are right, is awesome. Cleavage on demand rocks! A large chest can be a hypnotic tool that can make you the Pied Piper of seduction, and you don't have to resort to drastic measures to fill out the top half of a dress. A large chest can be considered womanly, feminine, and sexy.

Finding the right clothing that flatters your larger chest certainly has its own share of challenges, especially if you want to balance your look. So, my buxom beauties, let's give you some control over the situation, as you learn about the strategies that are right for you.

The three CASE strategies for you are Angle, Shape, and Elongate.

angle

▶ Deeper, angled necklines break up the space of your fuller chest, thereby balancing the fullness.

shape

▶ When you shape your waist through fitted and wrap tops, you balance the fullness of your bustline and avoid looking like a big buxom box.

elongate

▶ Wearing tops that are no shorter than two to three inches below your hipbone, which I refer to as the "hipbone zone," elongates your torso and balances the fullness of your bustline.

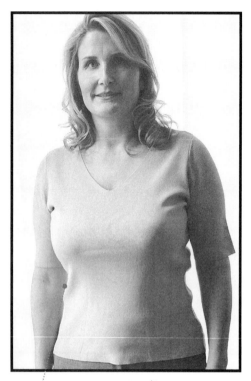

Big boobs are emphasized with a shorter, less-shaped top.

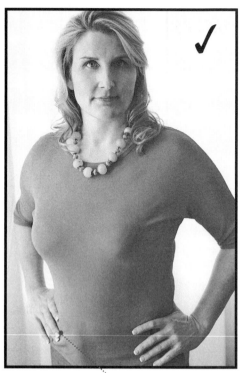

Big boobs are minimized and balanced with a longer, shaped top.

Most women with large chests never tuck their shirts into their pants because when they do, they look like they have boobs and a waist with no torso in between. One of the tricks to elongate the shortness of the torso that is created through having a larger chest is to add length to the hem of your shirt, which therefore elongates your torso and makes your bustline appear balanced.

In the photo on the left, our model's shirt is short with not much shape. Even her shapeless sleeves make her look more buxom, but not necessarily in a flattering way. This is because the shapeless shortness of her shirt shortens her torso and makes her boobs look bigger.

In the photo on the right, the model's shirt is slightly longer than the shirt she's wearing on the left, which balances her bustline.

There are a few key rules to applying this trick. First, the longer shirt you choose must have shape. If you wear a longer top without shape, then the fullness of your shirt falls straight from the fullness of your bustline, making you look heavier and as wide as your bust.

Second, you never want your shirt to be any shorter than your hipbones, and two to three inches below the hipbone is an ideal range for a shirt length. If you are petite with a larger chest, you can go a bit shorter, but it is still important that your shirt be at least as long as your hipbone point.

Many women put on shapeless tops thinking that they are camouflaging the largeness of their chests. These two photographs will show that this is not necessarily the case.

Women who have a large chest usually have a defined waist in comparison to the size of their chest. The biggest mistake you can make if you have a large chest is to bypass this slimmer part of your body. If you don't define your waist, you wind up looking as big and wide as the size of your chest. You also risk looking shorter and dumpier.

As evidenced in the photo on the left, our model looks much heavier and bustier in a top that has little to no shape, which makes her look very boxy and wide because her clearly defined waist is hidden.

In the photo on the right, you can see that while the neckline may be lower and revealing, the model looks slimmer, taller, and more balanced. This is because the top has shape in the waist.

You may also notice that the shaped shirt our model is wearing on the right makes her chest look more contained, whereas the shapeless top makes her chest look shapeless and uncontained. Don't let your boobs run free under a top that has no shape or structure.

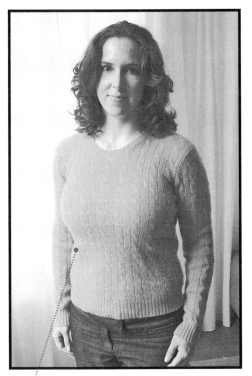

Big boobs are emphasized with a shapeless top.

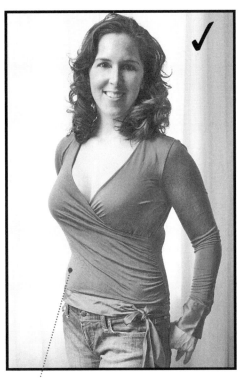

Big boobs are minimized with a shaped top.

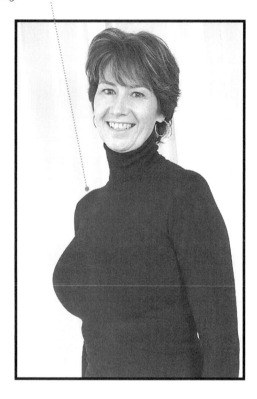

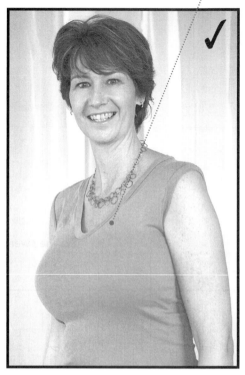

In the photo on the left, you can see how the higher neckline makes the fullness of the bustline look bigger than it already is and makes our model look top-heavy. With the unbroken space and less open neckline, it looks as if she is doing an ineffective job of hiding two bowling balls under a blanket, and her chest seems to begin somewhere below the neck.

When you add angles to an area of your body where you are fuller, you minimize its appearance, so the angled V-neck top that our model is wearing on the right minimizes her fuller chest. Additionally, the deeper neckline breaks up the space of her chest, which also creates a balancing and minimizing effect.

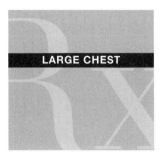

LARGE CHEST

- Choose deeper necklines.
- Shape your waist.
- Choose tops that hit at the "hipbone zone."

If you have a large chest . . .

- Replace your bras regularly. They wear out in about four to five months. The longer you wear your bras, the farther south your boobs are going to droop.

- In order to let your bras retain their elasticity, never wear the same bra two days in a row. Giving your bra a day to rest enables the Lycra or spandex to bounce back and revert to its original shape.

- Avoid chunky, heavy necklaces that hang over your boobs. Adding chunkier jewelry will just make your boobs look bigger. If you want to wear a necklace that is chunkier, choose styles that are shorter and don't lie over your chest.

- Don't buy tops, dresses, or jackets that have patch pockets, pocket flaps, or any other eye-catching details that lie right over your chest unless you want to say, "Look at my boobs!"

quick tips

Large Arms

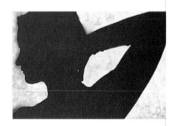

IF YOU HAVE large arms, you may be reluctant to leave the house in anything sleeveless without a coordinating sleeved component. You may also feel that there is a whole section of the clothing store—sans sleeves—that should be roped off. To you, leaving the house in something sleeveless is like asking you to walk out of the house naked.

To make matters worse, sleeves aren't always the magic solution to concealing larger arms. Have you ever tried on a shirt with sleeves that aren't large enough to fit around your arms? This works wonders on the self-esteem, doesn't it? There you are, stuffing your arm into a sleeve and feeling as if you are filling a sausage casing, convinced that you accidentally grabbed something from the children's department. Once you do finally get your arms into the sleeves, you fear that one false move may make you look like the Incredible Hulk after he loses his temper.

There are no surgical solutions to large arms, and you have probably found that exercise will tone a larger arm but will hardly whisk the excess completely away. So what's the solution? Is there really a way to get your arms out from hiding? Through the right clothing choices, you can be freed of your worries, and you can leave your house feeling great about your arms without completely covering them up. So instead of wearing long sleeves in ninety-degree weather and using a shawl as if it were a security blanket, let's explore the strategies developed specifically to get your arms out of hiding.

To balance fuller arms, there are three CASE strategies you can use: Angle, Shape, and Elongate.

angle

▶ Large arms look slimmer when capped off by a cap sleeve with an angled line, because angled and diagonal lines have a slimming effect.

shape

▶ Big bulky sleeves make large arms look big and bulky—you aren't hiding anything. Instead, choose sleeves that softly shape the arm area.

elongate

▶ Adding length to a full area slims it out. Wearing a fitted short sleeve with a bit of length that ends just above your elbow helps to elongate the area and make it look slimmer.

▶ Vertically striped sleeves elongate and slim a fuller arm because vertical lines are slimming. Horizontal stripes have a widening effect and shouldn't be found anywhere on a substantial arm.

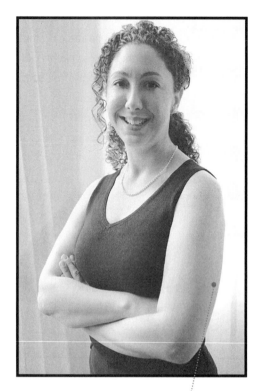 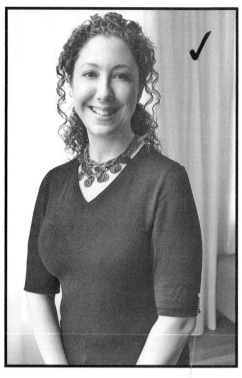

Large arms
look larger with
sleeveless
shirts.

Large arms look slim in shaped
short sleeves that are slightly
longer and end right above the elbow.

While you may leave home wearing sleeveless shirts, if you have large arms, going sleeveless isn't your first choice, and the photo on the left shows why.

Compare the photo on the left to the photo on the right: you can see just how much longer and leaner the arm looks in the photo on the right. When a larger arm is shaped by a short sleeve that has a bit of length, the sleeve elongates the fuller arm, and whenever you elongate an area, you also slim it.

It is important to note the type of short sleeve that helps create this effect. The one our model is wearing in the photo on the right isn't a dumpy wide sleeve that camouflages her arms. Instead, the sleeve shapes and elongates her arms by sitting close to them without clinging, making them look slimmer than any bulky sleeve ever could.

Wherever you place a vertical line on the body, it has a slimming and narrowing effect. Horizontal lines widen and make an area of the body look bigger than it is.

When it comes to having larger arms, knowing this rule can be the difference between your arms looking slimmer or fuller. The effects that vertical and horizontal lines have are clearly pictured here.

In the picture on the left, you can see that the horizontal stripes make our model's arms look wider and fuller.

In the picture on the right, our model is wearing a top that has vertical stripes. The vertical line of the sleeves creates an elongating effect that makes her arms look much slimmer.

When choosing stripe direction for fuller arms, always go vertical instead of horizontal. If vertical stripes aren't an option, then opt for no stripes at all.

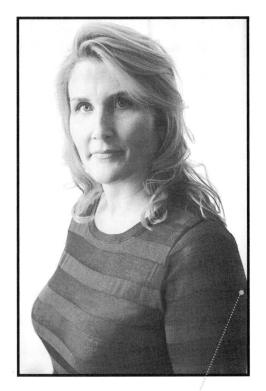

A fuller arm looks bigger with horizontal stripes.

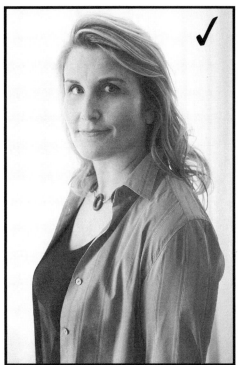

A fuller arm is slimmed with vertical stripes.

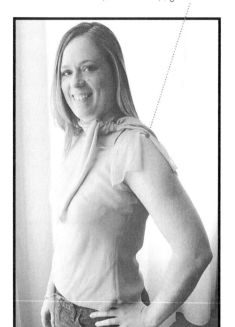

Large arms look bigger with a sloppy sleeve.

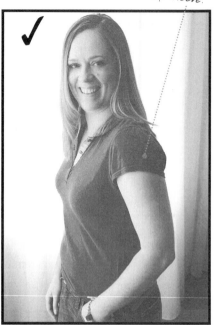

✔

Large arms look slimmer with an angled cap sleeve.

If you have large arms, it is all about the sleeves you choose. I've found that most women with large arms are often terrified of cap sleeves when in actuality cap sleeves are one of the most slimming sleeves you can choose. Why? Lines that angle have a slimming effect in any area that you place them on your body; therefore, in using the angle of the cap sleeve, your arms will look slimmer and less full.

In the picture on the left, our model is wearing a sleeve that splits right up the middle and exposes more of her arm, something you probably want to avoid. In addition, an area that is full needs the structure of a sleeve. When full areas aren't contained with some structure, they tend to jiggle and move more than you prefer.

There are some rules about choosing the right cap sleeve. The cap sleeve pictured on the right is one of the more flattering for a woman with large arms because it sits away from the arm yet still has some structure to it. When a cap sleeve sits away from a fuller arm, the arm looks naturally thinner in juxtaposition to the fuller width of the sleeve. Don't choose a cap sleeve that squeezes your arm or makes you look like you stuffed your arm into the sleeve. If the sleeve is too tight, your arm will spill out, making it look heavier—exactly what you're trying to avoid.

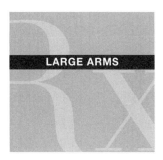

LARGE ARMS

- Use angled cap sleeves to slim the arm.
- Choose shaped sleeves.
- Use vertical stripes to slim the arm.

If your arms are large . . .

▪ If the sleeves of your favorite knits or sweaters are too tight, you can block and stretch out the sleeves. Wash the item, and while it's still damp, lay it down, stretch the width of the sleeves slightly, and allow the sweater or knit to dry flat.

▪ Scared of letting your arms go bare but still want to wear that sleeveless dress to an outdoor summer wedding? Try an overpiece with sheer sleeves: you'll have the illusion of bare arms while still feeling the protection of being covered up.

▪ Avoid too many bells and whistles, such as ruffles or bows, around your arm area. You are better off keeping this area free from too many distractions.

quick tips

Thin Arms

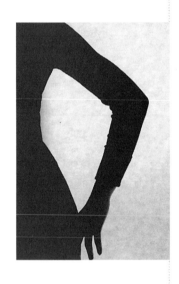

WHILE IT SEEMS that most women want to avoid oversized arms, you, on the other hand, would be quite happy if your arms were a bit less spindly. It isn't that you don't appreciate your fine limbs (being compared to Olive Oyl is certainly better than being compared to Popeye), but that doesn't mean that you don't have your own share of clothing problems.

Your arms may not fill out sleeves and may be barely large enough to fill the armhole of a tank top (leaving gaping views of your bra). Because a bangle bracelet wears more like a hula hoop than a piece of jewelry on your arm, with one quick flick of the wrist, you can fling it clear across a room.

Yes, you are aware that you would be considered the underdog at an arm-wrestling contest and have had your arms compared to a popular type of pasta. But this doesn't bother you. What does bother you, however, is not knowing the right clothes to choose to make your arms look fuller and more substantial. In this section, you'll learn how to balance, embrace, and make the best of your thinner arms.

The CASE strategies for you are Counterbalance, Shape, and Shorten.

counterbalance

▶ Avoid chunky, heavy bracelets, which will make your thin arms look skinnier than they already are. Instead, choose a finer and smaller bracelet, which will counterbalance your thinner upper arm and make it look fuller and more balanced.

shape

▶ Contrary to popular belief, shaping your thin arms by wearing a slimmer and more shaped sleeve makes your arms look bigger. Get rid of the big bell sleeves and sloppy, voluminous sleeves, which will only look like your arms are too thin to fill your shirt.

shorten

▶ Whenever you shorten an area, you also widen it. Horizontal lines have a shortening effect, which widens the arm. Wearing a sleeve with horizontal stripes will make your arm look fuller. Vertical lines and stripes have a slimming effect and will make your arms look thinner than they already are.

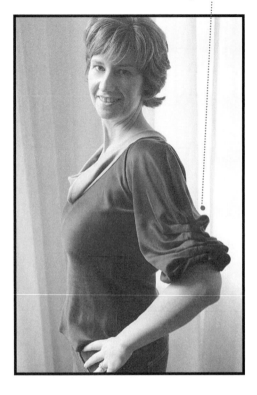

Thin arms look thinner in a bulky sleeve.

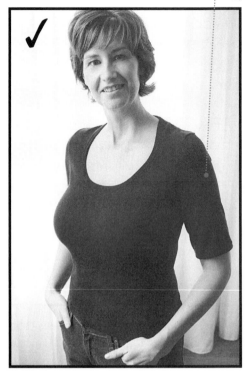

Thin arms look bigger with a slimmer sleeve.

It is common to want to bulk up a thin arm with a lot of fabric so that the full sleeve will make up for the areas where you are not so full. In fact, the opposite is true. In the photo on the left, you can see that all the excess fabric is spilling around her arm, as if it can't fill out her sleeve. As a result, her arm looks thinner and more spindly. Don't let the fabric pile up around your arms; shape your arms with slimmer sleeves instead.

If you look at our model in the picture on the right, in which she wears a slim, tapered sleeve, her arm actually looks bigger because she looks like she can fill out her sleeve.

When you put something big and bulky next to something very small and fine like a thinner arm, the largeness of that item makes anything next to it look even smaller. Looking at the photo on the left, you can see how a large and chunky bracelet next to her thin arm enhances the thinness of an area that is already quite slim. The chunkiness of the bangle bracelets overpowers her arms and makes them look even thinner.

In the photo on the right, our model is wearing a fine, delicate bracelet. Because the bracelet matches the fineness of her slimmer arms, her arm looks balanced and fuller.

When looking for a bracelet, the thinner your arms, the finer the bracelet you should choose. Also, go for a bracelet that isn't a bangle or too stiff and that can move and shape more to your wrist.

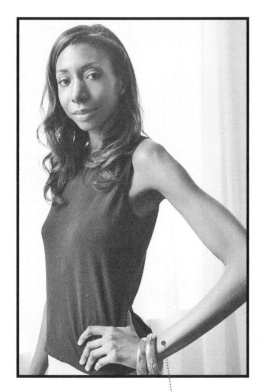

Thin arms look slimmer in a big, chunky bracelet.

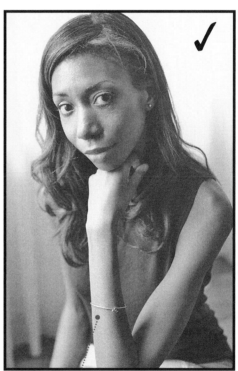

Thin arms look bigger with a finer bracelet.

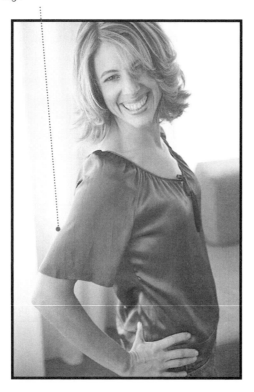

Thin arms look slimmer in big, wide sleeves.

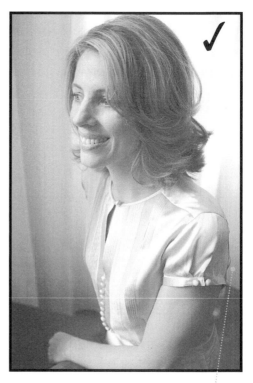

✓

Thin arms look bigger in puff sleeves.

In the photo on the left, the sleeve opening for our model is too wide, and poking out from the hem is a thin, spindly arm. With so much width, the arm looks even skinnier. It might seem logical to choose a big, bell sleeve for your thin arms, hoping that the fullness will hide the thinness, but you can see from this picture that this is not the case.

Looking at the photo on the right, you can see that the small puff is just enough to fill out a thin arm, without the fullness overwhelming the arm area and ultimately making it look thinner. The band at the hem of the sleeve contains the fullness, and the model's arm looks fuller.

If there is anyone who can wear a puff sleeve, it is someone who has a slim arm. The beauty of a puff sleeve for someone with a slimmer arm is that the puff is gathered and tighter at the bottom of the sleeve, and therefore the hem of the sleeve sits nicely against the arm. A word of caution, however: Make sure that the puff isn't too puffy. Not only will it be too overpowering for your slim arms, but you run the risk of looking juvenile. Also, if you have broad shoulders along with thin arms, an overly puffy sleeve will make your shoulders appear even broader.

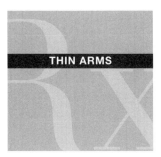

THIN ARMS

- Choose finer, thinner bracelets.
- Choose slim, narrow sleeves.
- Choose sleeves with horizontal stripes, not vertical ones.

If your arms are thin . . .

- You are someone who can get away with sleeve details such as ties, bows, and other attention-grabbing elements. This fullness and activity on your sleeves can also make your arms appear larger.

- Watch out for armholes that are too big in jackets and tops; the bigger the armhole, the bigger, wider, and fuller the sleeve will be. Go for finer knits, slim-fitting jackets, and tops that have a smaller and higher armhole.

- A tailor can taper the width of the sleeves on your jackets and shirts. When a jacket or shirt has sleeves that are too wide for your arms, you can appear shorter and as if your arms can't fill out your sleeves. This should be a last resort for you, as this type of tailoring can be costly, especially on a jacket that is lined.

quick tips

Long Arms

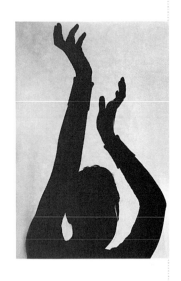

THERE ARE FEW things more frustrating than finding the perfect jacket and being faced with the following lose-lose situation: not buying it, or purchasing it and looking like Eddie Munster every time you wear it because the sleeves are just too short. If you have long arms, you understand this dilemma.

You also understand that a cuff that rolls back on a jacket or shirt is like a bonus of extra fabric that you can roll down so your sleeves actually fit. You know that three-quarter sleeves don't end midway up your forearm as they should and instead end uncomfortably right at your elbow. Long arms aren't just found on tall women; you can be petite with long arms, and while finding tops and jackets that are long enough for your arms may not be a problem, when you are petite, your arms may still look disproportionate to the rest of your body.

So while you may feel ready to put yourself into a straitjacket (not because of the struggle you have endured to find sleeves that are long enough, but because the sleeves on a strait-jacket may actually be long enough for you!), before committing yourself, check out the strategies in this section. You'll learn how to make your beautiful arms look more proportionate and balanced with the rest of your body.

The CASE method for long arms is to Shorten, and here's how:

shorten

▶ Avoid bracelet-length sleeves, which will make you look as if you grew out of them. A bracelet-length sleeve is one that is slightly shorter than a long sleeve but not short enough to be a true three-quarter sleeve.

▶ A cuff on a shirt will make your arms look shorter.

▶ Horizontal rather than vertical stripes on your sleeves make the arms look shorter.

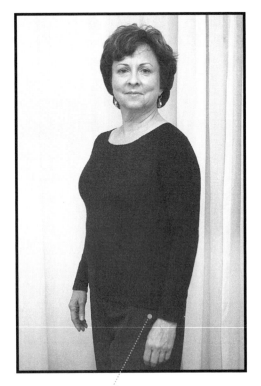

Long arms look longer without a cuff.

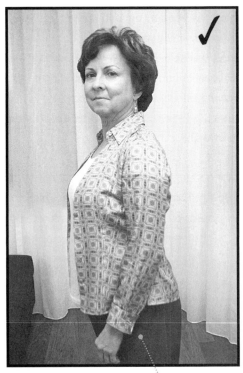

Long arms are shortened with a cuff.

Wherever you place a horizontal line on the body, that area will appear shorter. In the picture on the left, our model's arms look much longer without cuffs. If you have long arms, cuffs will always make your arms look shorter.

In the picture on the right, the cuff forms a shortening horizontal line, making the model's arms look shorter than in the picture on the left.

Horizontal lines placed anywhere on a body shorten that area, whereas vertical lines elongate an area. You can see the effects of shortening horizontal lines and elongating vertical lines in these two photos.

In the picture on the left, the vertical lines on our model's sleeves elongate her arms. While the sleeves are certainly long enough for her long arms, the vertical lines make her arms appear even longer than they already are. Even though her shirt has a cuff, which would normally shorten the look, it is because those vertical lines are so bold that they make her arms look even longer. You can see how long her arms are naturally: notice where her thumb knuckles are in relationship to where her crotch is.

In the picture on the right, the horizontal lines on the sleeves make our model's arms appear shorter and more in proportion to her body. Even though the sleeves are on the shorter side, the horizontal stripes throughout make that shorter sleeve work.

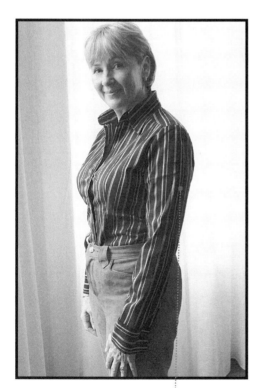

Arms appear longer with vertical stripes on the sleeve.

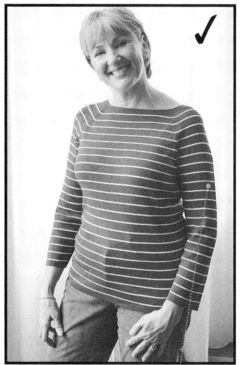

Arms appear shorter with horizontal stripes on the sleeve.

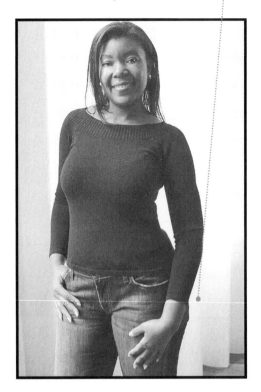

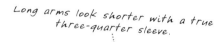

With long arms, it is hard to find any long-sleeve shirt that doesn't make you look like you outgrew the sleeves. There may be few sleeves out there that are perfect for you, but there certainly are some options that are better than others.

The term three-quarter sleeve is pretty broad. It seems that a three-quarter sleeve can hit at any point on the forearm. When you have long arms, it is important to choose the most suitable three-quarter sleeve or else you may be overemphasizing the length of your arms.

Look at the picture on the left. This type of sleeve would be considered a bracelet length. It's not a full-length sleeve, but it isn't really short enough to be called a three-quarter sleeve either.

Because it looks like the sleeves simply aren't long enough for our model, this is an awkward length for her, and her arms look longer.

In the picture on the right, our model is wearing what we would refer to as a true three-quarter sleeve. Her sleeve ends only a few inches below her elbow. Even though she has long arms, she doesn't look like she outgrew her sleeves because the sleeve looks like it should end at the point where it does.

Whenever you don't want to emphasize the length of your arms, find a three-quarter sleeve that ends right below your elbow; anything longer will just look like your sleeves aren't long enough or that they shrank in the wash.

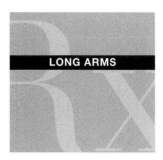

LONG ARMS

- Wear true three-quarter sleeves.
- Use cuffs to shorten arms.
- Choose sleeves with horizontal stripes.

If your arms are long . . .

- The sleeves on your knits and sweaters can be stretched a bit to compensate for your longer arms. While a washed sweater is still damp, stretch the sleeves vertically and allow to dry flat.

- Bigger bracelets and watches fill in the space between your hand and your sleeve, so you don't look like you outgrew your sleeves. If your sleeves are too short, fill in the spaces with bigger accessories around your wrists.

- Cropped pants emphasize your longer arms. You don't have to eliminate them from your wardrobe, but avoid wearing cropped pants and cropped sleeves at the same time, which will really emphasize how long your arms are.

Short Waist

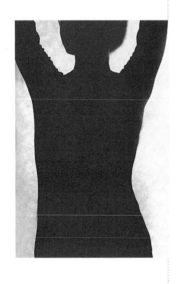

IF YOU HAVE a short waist, you may wonder if your body was built from mismatched parts in the leftover bin, as your squat top half isn't in proportion to the much longer bottom half of your body. While the rest of the world may envy your long legs, you feel like a flamingo — hardly consolation for not having a torso. In fact, it feels like your boobs rest comfortably at your waistline and that your waist seems to begin somewhere around your armpits.

Being short-waisted comes equipped with its own dressing challenges. You may have to constantly shorten long straps on tank tops, and most dresses are out of the question because your own waist is located inches above the waistline of the dress. You wouldn't dare tuck a shirt into your pants, there isn't a belt to be found in your wardrobe, and most T-shirts are too long for you.

Your frustrations with being squat in the middle may have gotten so extreme that you have considered volunteering yourself as the rope in a game of tug-of-war. But there's hope. You'll be happy to know that you don't have to maintain the posture of a prima ballerina to make it seem like you have a longer torso. With the strategies in this section, you'll learn how to choose clothing that will make your top and bottom halves appear like a perfectly matching set.

The CASE strategy for a short waist is to elongate it. Here's how:

elongate

▶ Bypass the waist altogether with longer jackets. The longer jacket elongates and pulls the attention away from how short your waist is.

▶ Wear a jacket over a monochromatic shirt and bottom. The uniform color creates a longer-looking torso. If the jacket is in a brighter and more eye-catching shade than your pants and shirt, it will also detract from your waist.

▶ Wearing low-rise pants will elongate the look of your torso.

▶ Because vertical lines elongate, stripes or ribbing on a sweater create an illusion of a longer torso.

▶ Avoid cropped shirts, cropped jackets, or shirts that are shorter than your hipbone; your top half will look squat and your bottom half longer—exactly what we are trying to avoid. Choose tops that hit your hipbone or are in the two- to three-inch "hipbone zone."

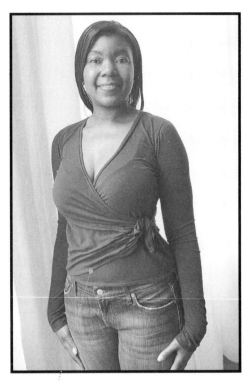

*A short waist is
shortened with a
shorter top.*

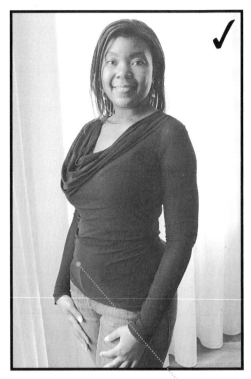

*A short waist is
elongated with a
longer shirt.*

The shorter your shirt is, the squatter your torso is going to look. In the photo on the left, the top half of our model's body looks short, squat, and out of proportion to the longer lower half of her body. In addition, the shirt is a wrap style, and all that activity in her midsection is cutting her off and making her look even squatter.

In the photo on the right, you can see that our model's shirt is within the two- to three-inch hipbone zone range. Because of this, the top half of her body looks elongated and in propor-tion to the rest of her body. When you have a shorter waist, many of the shirts you try on are going to be long on you, but it is important that the tops are not too long, especially if you are petite, which is why the "hipbone zone" meas-urement is so helpful.

When choosing tops, try to keep them shaped in the waist and within that hipbone zone. Also try to avoid too much horizontal distraction—such as ties and wraps—at your midsection.

Horizontal lines have a shortening effect on the body wherever they are placed; vertical lines have a lengthening effect. So when it comes to an area of your body where you would like to see more length, stay away from horizontal lines!

These photos say it perfectly. In the photo on the left, the horizontal lines in the jacket shorten her already short torso, making her look squat and short on top. Does this mean that you must swear off horizontally striped shirts for good? Not at all, but be careful of the ones you choose. If you would like to wear horizontal stripes, never buy a horizontally striped shirt that is cropped or shorter than your hipbone zone, and always make sure that the shirt you choose has shape and isn't boxy and wide. Boxy, wide shirts will make you look even shorter-waisted because the wide boxiness of the top or jacket creates even more of a shortening effect.

In the photo on the right, our model is wearing a vertically striped shirt. These stripes create the look of a longer torso because they force the eye to see more length, which balances out the visual shortness of her torso. It is easy to see how much longer her torso looks compared to how it looks in the photo on the left.

A shorter waist is shortened with horizontal lines.

A shorter waist is elongated with vertical lines.

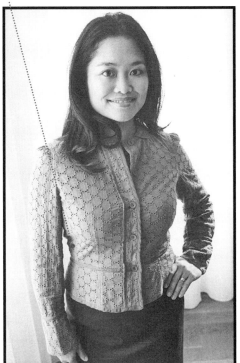

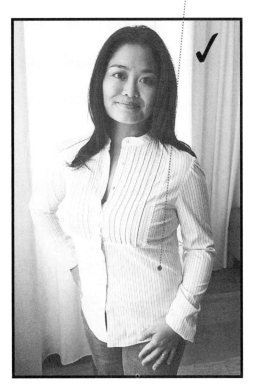

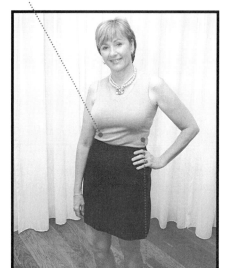

A short waist is shortened through tucking in.

A short waist is shortened when the natural waist is defined.

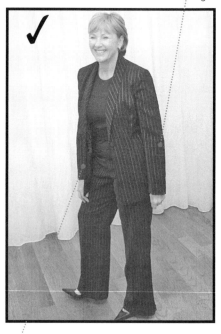

A short waist is elongated through monochromatic dressing.

A short waist is elongated with a longer jacket that bypasses the waist.

One of the best things you can do when you have a short waist is not to call attention to it. The biggest no-no for a short waist is tucking in, which you can clearly see in the photo on the left. When you tuck in, you call attention to where your naturally short waist is located. Also, because her top is so much lighter in color than her skirt, we can clearly see where her waist is located and how short it is. She could have saved this outfit by adding a longer jacket over the light-colored top and darker skirt, which would elongate the waist by bypassing it just like the jacket is doing in the photo on the right. Another solution would have been not to tuck in

the shirt, or at least to have the top and the skirt be closer in color.

In the picture on the right, the outfit worn by our model draws the attention away from the fact that her waist is short, for two reasons. First, the longer jacket bypasses the waist, and so your eye sees the length of the jacket rather than the shortness of her waist. Second, with the monochromatic coloring of the shirt and pants, there is no color change at the waistline, which would create a horizontal line. Her shorter waist isn't defined, and our model looks like she has a longer, more proportioned torso.

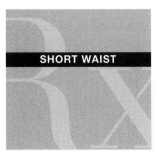

SHORT WAIST

- Choose drop-waisted tops.
- Bypass the waist with longer jackets.
- Choose monochromatic outfits.
- Wear low-rise pants.
- Wear vertically striped tops.
- Choose hipbone-zone tops.

quick tips

If your waist is short . . .

- If your knit shirt isn't long enough and is making you look squat, try to double-layer a longer top under the shorter one to create an overall longer look.

- Avoid belts whenever possible, and never wear a belt that doesn't match the color of your pants; this only creates a glaring horizontal line that says, "Look how short my waist is."

- A skinnier belt is always a better choice than a wide belt. A wide belt takes up more space in your torso area and only makes your waist look shorter.

Long Waist

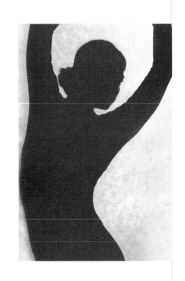

WHILE IT MAY seem like a medical mystery and that you have a few extra vertebrae, it's not and you don't: You simply have a long waist. Like your girlfriends with short waists, you feel that your top half and bottom half are a mismatched set. In addition, your legs probably feel like imposters: two short, dinky appendages trying to pass themselves off as the real thing, because when you get right down to it, you are all torso.

Sound familiar?

Maybe you think you need Crazy Glue or a staple gun to keep your shirts tucked into the back of your pants (in fact, in moments of desperation, you've actually considered it). *Painful* is the word you use to describe what it feels like to wear a one-piece bathing suit as you constantly dig it out of the crack of your bum. Baring your stomach isn't a choice—instead, it's more of an inevitability. And while the rest of the female population picketed against low-rise pants, you admitted to liking them.

Even if you're tall, with a long waist, you may have been spotted perusing the petite department for a pair of pants because your legs are so short in relation to your torso.

There is hope for those of you who have been endearingly called "top-tall" and wish that your torso came equipped with its own retractable feature. With the strategies in this section, you will be given clothing solutions needed to make your long torso a little less lanky and your look a little more balanced.

The best CASE method for a long waist is to shorten it. Here's how:

shorten

▶ Belt longer tops at your waist with a belt or scarf, which will shorten your long torso area by adding an attention-grabbing horizontal line (which, as you know, has a shortening effect). Select a belt that is brightly colored or contrasts with your pants to further break up the length.

▶ Horizontally striped shirts shorten your torso for the same reason. Vertical lines have the opposite effect, so avoid vertical stripes, seams, or ribbed knits on top.

▶ You can also break up the length of your torso with a cropped jacket or shrug.

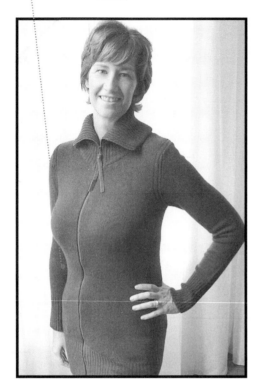

A long waist is elongated with a tunic.

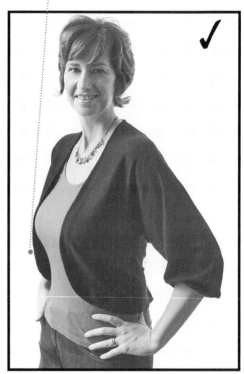

A long waist is shortened with a cropped jacket.

✓

The more you break up the length of your torso with horizontal lines, the shorter your waist will appear. In the photo on the left, our model is wearing a long sweater tunic, and there is no horizontal line breaking up her torso; therefore, her torso looks longer. Because there are no shortening horizontals at her torso, the eye is forced to see length. Additionally, vertical lines elongate, so the vertical line of the zipper creates an elongating line, making her torso look even longer.

In the photo on the right, the cropped jacket shortens our model's waist because the horizontal line created by the jacket breaks up the space.

Tunic tops are not the most flattering for women with long torsos because the longer the top, the longer your torso will look—and the shorter your legs will look as well. In many cases, having a long torso means that you also have short legs, and the last thing you want to do is make your legs appear shorter with such a long top. A better choice is a longer top that doesn't hang below your crotch point. This is also the case for longer jackets; unless you have a longer torso that also includes long legs, you are better off keeping your jackets on the shorter side.

If you have a long waist or long torso, no matter what top you wear, it is usually pretty obvious that your waist is long. But by simply belting your top around the waist, the horizontal line of the belt breaks up the length of your waist, thereby shortening it. Remember, horizontal lines anywhere on the body shorten that area.

The photographs below show our model in the same turtleneck. In the photograph on the left, she appears without a belt, and you can see that when the eye isn't stopped by a belt, her

waist looks longer. In our model's case, she successfully shortens her waist with a belt that matches the color of her top, but if you really want to break up your longer torso with a belt, opt for a contrasting belt color that will really stand out.

There is one caution with this solution: You may want to avoid a belt if you have a larger chest. A larger chest already has its own torso-shortening effect, and adding the belt at your waist may increase the visual size of your chest.

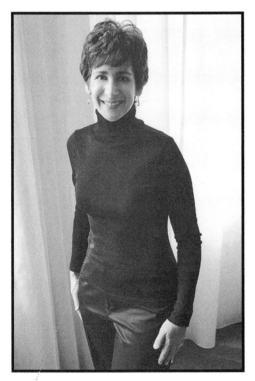

A long waist looks long without a belt.

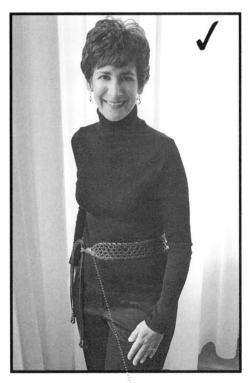

A long waist is shortened with a belt.

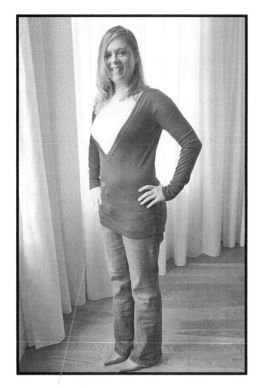

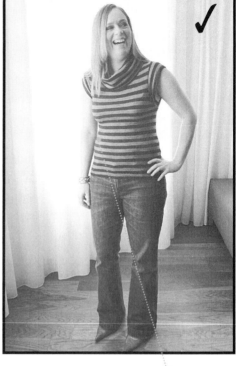

A long waist is
elongated without
horizontal stripes.

A long waist is
shortened with
horizontal stripes.

In the photo on the left, you can see that a long tunic elongates our model's long waist. Additionally, the plunging depth of the V-neck diverts the eyes downward, causing you to see even more length. If you have a long waist, and a long tunic-style top is something you are going to consider, try one without such a deep neckline. Also consider a wider rib at the bottom of the tunic, which will have a shortening effect on the longer sweater style.

You can see in the photo on the right that our model's torso looks shorter because of the horizontal stripes she is wearing. However, while horizontal lines can have a shortening effect, they can also have a widening effect. If you tend to gain weight in your midsection or are aware that horizontal stripes do make you look wider, use this strategy with caution and choose horizontally striped tops that aren't too boxy and shape you more in your waist.

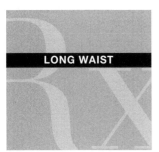

LONG WAIST

- Belt your tops.
- Choose contrasting colored belts.
- Wear horizontally striped tops.
- Wear shorter, cropped jackets over your tops.

If your waist is long . . .

- Choose thicker belts over skinny ones. A wider belt shortens your waist by creating a thicker, shortening horizontal. A skinnier belt will not have as great of an effect.

- To really cut the length of your torso, choose a belt that contrasts in color to the outfit you are wearing. You are someone who can wear a brightly colored belt in a pop color really well.

- Avoid tops with too much Lycra or spandex if you want to keep your T-shirts from popping up and exposing your midriff. Lycra or spandex has a spring effect, which can keep your shirts from staying put.

- Even though your shirts say that they can be put in the dryer, choose to air-dry them instead. Heat from dryers will shrink and therefore shorten shirts after a few tumbles. If you must pop your shirts in the dryer, air-dry them as long as you can and then fluff them up at a cooler temperature.

quick tips

Slight Waist

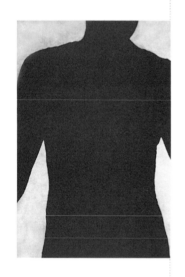

SOME WOMEN WANT to minimize their curves, but not you. Your lack of indentation at your waistline makes you feel more like the uncurvy number eleven rather than a womanly number eight.

Because of the lack of whittled definition between your waist and your hips, pants are in constant danger of falling down. You may have to let the waist out on your pants and skirts, and clothing without any shape in the waist can make you look like you're wearing a pillowcase. Drastic measures to fake a waist may have included tightening your belt a few notches extra to create an illusion of what isn't there, or purchasing clingy tops with so much spandex that they resemble scuba gear.

However, it doesn't take a gazillion repetitions of dizzying side bends to get a sculpted midsection, nor do you need to squeeze your waist like a tube of toothpaste either. All it takes is learning the best strategies and choosing the clothing that will give you the soft curves and voluptuousness you've been dying for.

Your CASE strategies for balancing a slight waist are Angle, Shape, and Elongate.

angle

▶ Shirts with diagonal lines like stripes or ribs create slimming angles and can slim the thickness of your waist.

▶ Pockets that angle on your jackets create slimming diagonal lines at your waist and make it look slimmer.

shape

▶ Wrap or corseted tops shape your waist area and create an illusion of what isn't there naturally—a waist.

▶ Baggy shapeless tops only emphasize that you have no waist. Shaped tops are a better choice because they help you define a waistline that you may not naturally have.

▶ Choose jackets with shape. Avoid shapeless jackets with no waist definition. The more shape, the more of a waist you will appear to have.

▶ Dresses with a defined waist are always a better choice than a shapeless dress with no defined waistline.

▶ Choose tops and jackets with princess seams, which are fitted seams that not only shape the waist area but also create the look of a more defined waist.

elongate

▶ Choose a single-breasted jacket over a double-breasted one whenever possible. Because of the optical width created by a double row of buttons in a double-breasted jacket, your waist looks wider than it already is.

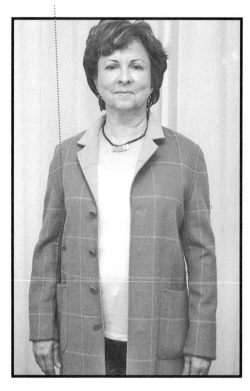

A slight waist looks undefined and shapeless in a jacket with no shape.

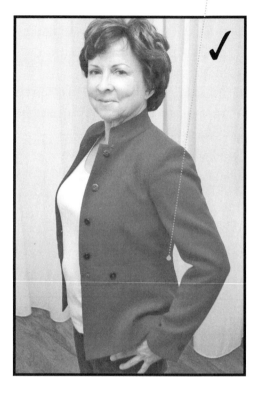

A slight waist looks more defined in a shaped jacket.

When choosing a jacket, coat, sweater, blouse, or T-shirt, I want you to remember what is going on in these two photographs. In the picture on the left, our model looks shapeless because she is wearing a jacket that has no shape. When you have no waist, instead of trying to hide it through shapeless clothing, use the power of shape to give yourself the body you want. Shapeless styles only make you look shapeless.

Because of the shaping of the jacket in the photo on the right, our model appears to have a much more shaped and defined waist. And by forcing the eye to see shape where she doesn't have it naturally, she also looks about ten pounds lighter. What a bonus!

Also notice that the shaped jacket on the right focuses attention on her shoulders and her face, versus the jacket on the left, which focuses attention on her midsection—just the part of the body she is trying not to call attention to.

In the photo on the left, our model looks as shapeless as the dress is. Because she doesn't have any shape through her waist, she looks short and squat in addition to having a shapeless waist.

While horizontal lines often widen an area on the body, it is important to note the benefit of the particular defined horizontal line in the photo on the right. The dress has a full skirt, and the waist is the most shaped part of the body and much more defined. Because of the balanced shape created by the dress, our model has a more balanced-looking body. Also notice that the belt is not cinched and pulled within an inch of its life. All it took was placing a belt at her waistline and partnering it with a fuller skirt to create a curvier figure.

Slimming out an area with shape also helps you appear taller, and you can see how much taller our model looks in the picture on the right than she does on the left.

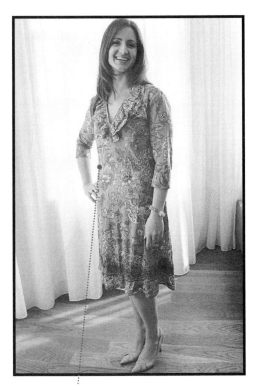

A slight waist looks even slighter in a dress without shape.

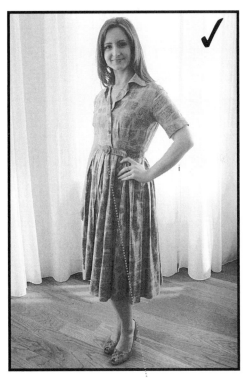

A slight waist looks more defined with a defined waistline.

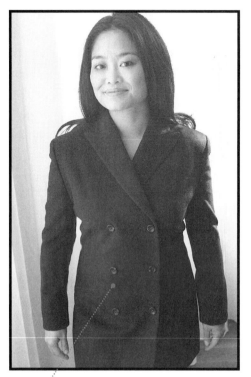

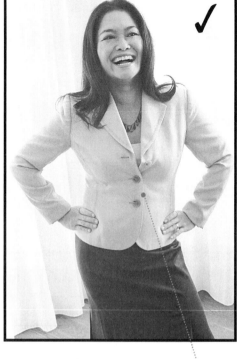

A slight waist is enhanced with a double-breasted jacket.

A slight waist is defined with a single-breasted jacket.

Double-breasted jackets are never a wise choice for someone who doesn't have much of a defined waist, and the photo on the left shows why. Just because the double-breasted jacket has two rows of vertical lines (and vertical lines do slim) does not mean that she looks doubly thinner. Because of the two sets of buttons that run up and down her body in a parallel manner, your eye is drawn more to the width between the two rows, making her waist look wider. The wider you set a row of double-breasted buttons apart, the wider and squarer your waist will look, so if you must wear a double-breasted jacket, be sure to choose one in which the two rows of buttons are closer to each other.

In the picture on the right, the single row of buttons on the jacket creates a slimming vertical line right down the middle of the model's body. Vertical lines always define an area and make it look slimmer.

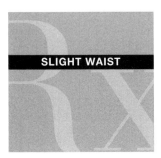

SLIGHT WAIST

- Add angles at your waist.
- Choose tops and jackets with shape.
- Wear dresses with definition in the waist.
- Choose single-breasted over double-breasted jackets.

If you have a slight waist . . .

- Shirts without shape can be taken to a tailor to have more definition created in the waist area.

- If you purchase a pair of pants that are too tight because they have a thicker or straighter waist area, see if there is a center back outlet—extra fabric in the waist area of the back—that allows for the waist to be let out. More expensive pants usually have a center back outlet. If you aren't sure if your pants have one, check with your tailor, who will know what to look for.

- If you are going to wear a belt, match it to the clothing you are wearing. A pop color or contrasting belt, even though it will cinch your waist, will also draw attention to it. Keep the loudness of your belt colors to a dull roar.

quick tips

Tummy

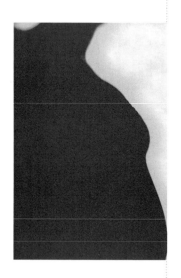

AS YOU TURN to the side and look in the mirror, there it is staring back at you: your tummy. Maybe you have a term for it, like your "pooch" or your "Buddha belly." (Heck, if it is going to be a lifelong companion, you may as well give it an endearing name.)

Or perhaps you never had a tummy until you bore children and then, like an elastic band that got overstretched, your tummy stayed looser, never bouncing back to it's pre-baby flatness.

Sure, you have considered a tummy tuck, have a girdle in your dresser, are willing to suspend all logic and believe that there really are panties out there promising to flatten out the bulge, and have wondered if breathing is really that important anyway. However, in the end, you finally resigned yourself to the possibility that your stomach will always be the body feature that gives you the most frustration.

You could spend the rest of your life sucking it in, never leaving the house without some sort of girdle, and assume that baggy, shapeless clothing is your only option. However, there is a way to get dressed and be able to exhale at the same time, and there are clothing choices and strategies for you that are both stylish and balancing. So stop sucking it in, exhale, and check out the strategies designed just for you.

The CASE strategies for a tummy are Angle and Shape.

angle

▶ Diagonal lines are slimming angles. Diagonal stripes on a top, jacket, or sweater minimize the tummy and make the area look slimmer.

shape

▶ A shirt that has gathering, or ruching, shapes and contours the tummy area and makes it hard to tell if it is your tummy or the gathering that is causing the bunching.

▶ Shirts, sweaters, and tops with shape cover up the tummy area by containing it and creating the look of a slimmer midsection.

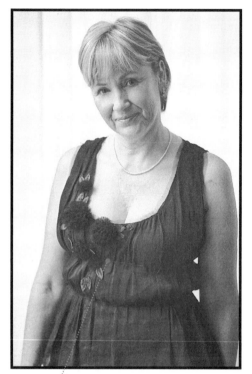

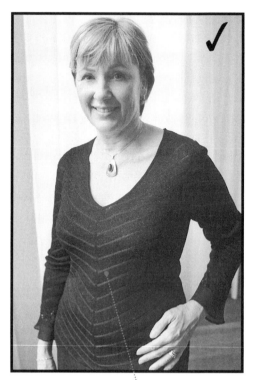

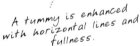
A tummy is enhanced
with horizontal lines and
fullness.

A tummy
is slimmed with
diagonal stripes.

Lines that angle or move in a diagonal fashion have a slimming effect, and you can see them in action here. In the photo on the left, several things are going on with this top that make it unflattering. First, horizontal lines can widen an area, and you can see that the horizontal lines that form the gathering on this top make her look wider and give her less shape. Additionally, while gathering can often do a good job of covering up what you want to hide, in this case it isn't working. Gathering in a top needs to have a lot of shape to work. Here, the gathering is creating fullness and an uncontained look in her tummy area.

In the photo on the right, even though the stripes of this sweater are black on black and not overly obvious, see how much slimmer she looks because of the slimming diagonal lines right over her tummy area.

Oftentimes many women with a tummy think that if they just hide out under layers of gathers, they will look slimmer. The truth is the opposite. This is why elastic-waist pants make a tummy look bigger and rounder. Areas of fullness do better when they are shaped and more contained, not covered up by a massive amount of gathers.

This model is a mother of two children. She didn't start out with a tummy naturally, but after having the area stretched through childbearing, she suddenly found her tummy to be an area of concern. Looking at the photo on the left, you can see that the shirt she is wearing is flimsy and not substantial enough to contain the softness of her tummy. As a result, you can see it is her tummy that is causing the slight bulge over her pants, often referred to as the muffin top.

One of the best strategies for an overelasticized tummy zone is to shape it with a top that has well-fitting gathers, also known as ruching. Unlike our model on the previous page, who wore a billowy gathered top, the shape in the shirt that our model is wearing on the right acts in a way that contains her stomach, and shaped gathers camouflage and make it impossible to tell what is causing the bunching—her stomach or the way the shirt is constructed.

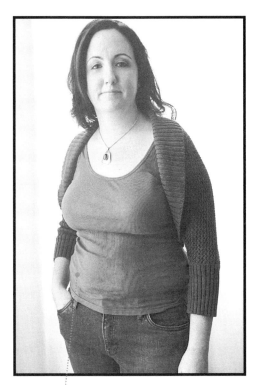

A tummy looks bigger in tops that are too thin and can't contain the tummy.

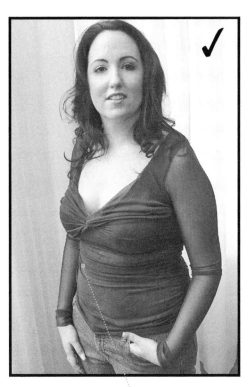

A tummy is minimized with shaped gathers and ruching.

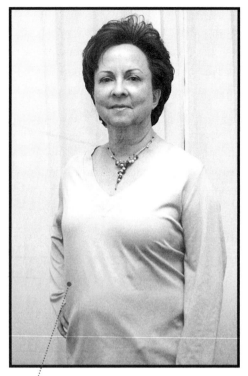

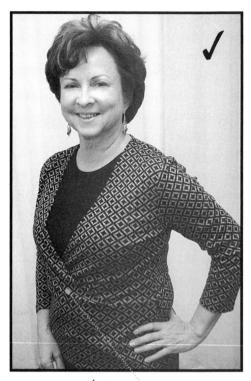

A tummy looks bigger in shapeless tops.

A tummy is minimized in shaped tops.

Have you ever gotten thoroughly discouraged by the size of your tummy and figured that if you just hid out under a shapeless top, nobody would ever know it was there? Well, as the pictures on this page can show you, the exact opposite is true.

In the photo on the left, while our model is clearly covering up something, it is pretty obvious what it is: her tummy. Instead of having a balanced shape and a defined waist, she just looks like a lumpy bag of bulges.

In the picture on the right, you can clearly see the power of shape. By wearing a shaped top, she doesn't look like she is trying to cover anything up; she is creating the shape she wants. Additionally, the wrap style of this top creates a slimming angle. Angles or lines that move in a diagonal fashion always slim an area that is fuller.

The next time you go to grab your tent of a tunic to cover your tummy, remember the effect it is creating. Parts of the body that are fuller and softer need to be contained rather than running free under clothing that is loose and shapeless.

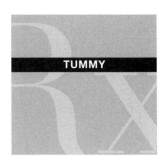

- Choose tops with angled lines.
- Use contained ruching or gathering to hide a tummy.
- Avoid shapeless tops.

If you have a tummy . . .

■ Fabrics with stretch in them are a real asset for you. Just make sure that the fabric is substantial enough in weight and heft, or it won't be heavy enough to contain your tummy.

■ Shaped does not mean skin-clinging. Avoid pants and tops that sit too close and tight to your body, or every lump and bulge will be visible.

■ Leave the pleated pants in the last decade; pleats, gathers, elasticized waists, and other fullness in your pants or skirts will just make your tummy look fuller and bumpier. Keep the front of your pants and skirts flat and free of any lumps and bumps.

Wide Hips

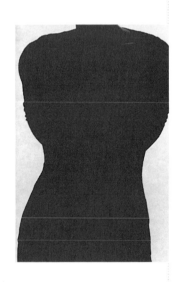

HUNDREDS OF YEARS ago, wide hips on a woman were a sign of health and fertility and a feature prized by their owners, as well as many men! Fast-forward a few hundred years to today: Femininity and fertility are still associated with the width of a woman's hips, yet you're not exactly feeling "owner love." Taking a job as a professional breeder isn't at the top of your dream-job list, and all your wide hips mean to you is that you look like a hula dancer when trying on a pair of pants.

Even more challenging is trying to find pants that have enough room to fit your shapely hips. Your hips may make you feel dumpy or bottom heavy, and while tight pants are uncomfortable, shapeless clothing only emphasizes the width of your hips, and too much shape in your clothing makes you feel like a bowling pin.

And no one's immune—whether you're a gamine nymph or a zaftig beauty, you can have wide hips. The width of your hips has more to do with your skeletal build than it does with the weight you carry in that region of your body. Therefore, as with most body issues, wishing or trying to exercise this feature away may ultimately feel like a fruitless effort. However, this news doesn't mean you have to spend the rest of your life feeling like John Wayne slinging two gun holsters at each side. By applying the right strategies, you will learn how to embrace and balance this womanly feature.

This common area of complaint can benefit from all the CASE strategies.

counterbalance

▸ Wider necklines counterbalance wider hips by adding opposing fullness at your neckline, which slims the appearance of your hips.

▸ Boot-cut pants or a fit-and-flare skirt counterbalances wider thighs by adding fullness at the opposite end of your body.

angle

▸ Diagonal lines create a slimming effect when applied to any part of the body that is wide or full. Skirts with diagonal stripes or lines that move on an angle will narrow your wider hips.

▸ Shirts with a shirttail hem create angles and taper your hip area. Conversely, shirts with a hem that cuts straight across horizontally and ends at the widest point of your hips create a widening effect of the hip area.

shape

▸ Shaping the waist creates a more balanced body shape. Shapeless jackets just make you look like a block as wide as your hip area.

▸ Stiff A-lines and shapeless skirts make you look shapeless and dumpy. Instead, choose a skirt that tapers slightly at the hem, also called a pegged or tapered skirt, which will make you look longer and leaner in the hips.

elongate

▸ Vertical lines always elongate an area that is wide, and when you elongate the hips, you also slim the area. Add vertical lines in your hip area through pinstripes, vertical seams, or a vertical row of buttons down the lower half of your body on your pants or skirts.

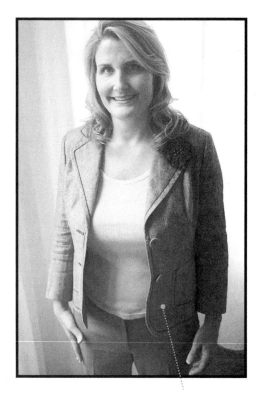

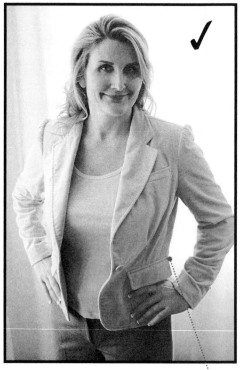

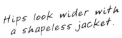

Hips look wider with a shapeless jacket.

Hips look slimmer with a shaped jacket.

When a woman has wide hips, most times she has a defined waist. By not emphasizing your waist and wearing jackets or tops that don't have shape in the waist area, you wind up bypassing one of the more flattering areas of your body and ultimately looking as wide as your hips.

In the photo on the left, our model's jacket has little to no shape. As a result, a straight line is created from her bustline to her hips, making her look boxy and as wide as her hips.

You can see in the photo on the right that the shape in the jacket creates more of a balanced body shape. Our model has a slimmer waist and therefore her body looks more balanced in a jacket that defines her waist.

Don't pass up the benefit of a defined waist when your hips are wide. Shapeless tops and jackets will only emphasize what you would rather camouflage.

Many women who have large hips think that if they cover them with shapeless skirts, nobody will know what is hiding underneath. While this tactic sometimes works, when it fails, it fails miserably.

Wide, shapeless skirts often make women with large hips just look wide and shapeless. In the picture on the left, you can see what a skirt with no shape or taper does to a wide hip. It looks like our model is wearing a large square for a skirt, and as a result, the lower half of her body looks squarer, heavier, and wider.

I know the idea of shaping your wider hips seems scary, but you can see that the skirt on the right, which slightly tapers and narrows at the hem (called a pegged hem), gives our model a more elongated and slimmer look. Additionally, the diagonal stripes in this skirt further taper and narrow her hips because diagonal lines or lines that angle always create a slimming effect.

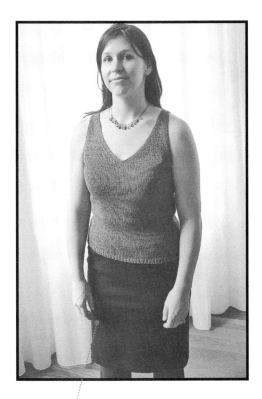

Wide hips look wider in square, straight skirts.

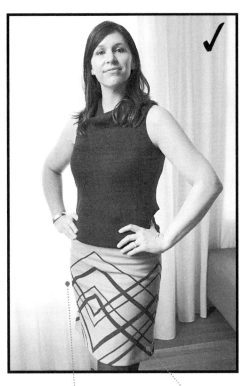

Wide hips are slimmed with diagonal lines.

Wide hips look narrower in a skirt that tapers at the hem.

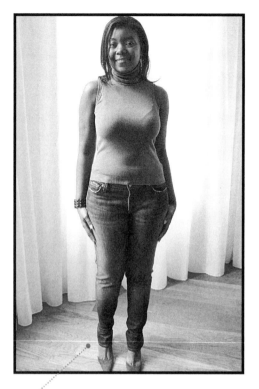

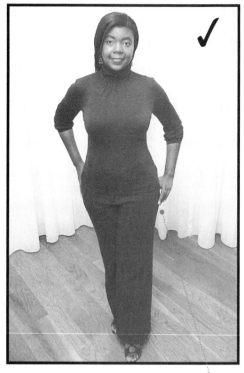

Wide hips look wider in pants that taper at the hem.

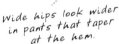

Wide hips look slimmer in pants that hang straight from the widest point of the hip.

In the photo on the left, you can see what happens when you put tapered pants on large hips. All they do is emphasize the width of the model's hip area by creating such a contrast between the narrowness at her hem and the width of her hips. As a result, all the attention is now on her hip area, emphasizing that it is the widest part of her body. Additionally, the sleeveless top isn't helping. Because the armhole cuts inward, it makes her hips look wider. Instead, a top with a wider neckline would have had positive counterbalancing effects because of the width created at her shoulders.

While the advice to wear pants that hang straight from the hip seems to be the opposite of the advice I just gave you about skirts, you can see in the photo on the right that the straight line of the pants from her hips does in fact elongate and camouflage the width of her hips, therefore making them look slimmer.

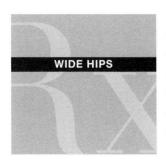

WIDE HIPS

- Wear wider necklines.
- Wear pants that fall straight from the hip.
- Choose boot-cut pants and fit-and-flare skirts.
- Wear tapered skirts.
- Angles and vertical lines slim the hips.
- Wear shaped jackets and tops.

If you have wide hips . . .

■ If you have a problem with your pockets popping open when you wear flat-front pants, have a tailor remove the pocket bags and stitch the pockets closed. Chances are there is little you can fit in the pockets of flat-front pants anyway.

■ Not sure if a pair of pants or a skirt has a pegged or tapered hem? While pants are still on the hanger, fold the hem of the pant leg back on itself to about where the knee would be—approximately twelve inches below the crotch. If the hem of the pant leg is wider than the knee of the pant leg, then the pants are more of a boot-cut style. If the width of the hem is as wide as the knee, then it is a straight-leg pant. And if the hem is narrower than the knee, then it is a pegged pant and should be avoided by anyone with wide hips. For skirts, you just have to fold the skirt back slightly on itself. If the skirt's hem is narrower than the body of the skirt, then it is a pegged skirt. If it is the same width or wider, the skirt doesn't peg or taper, and you may look a bit boxy and wide.

Narrow Hips

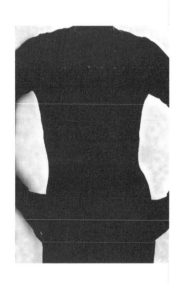

THE FEATURE MOST women today seem to covet? Narrow hips. With narrow hips, you have a long, lean line without too much curve getting in the way. Pants seem to glide on as if your thighs were presprayed with WD-40, and you can wear low-rise pants with little risk of anything additional spilling over, not to mention you may be blessed with relatively shapely and thin legs.

However, while most women would love to be a bit narrower in the hip, you know that with little curve from waist to hip, being boyishly narrow isn't the picnic it's cracked up to be. Often the narrowness of your hip area throws off the balance of the rest of your body, making your top half look proportionately broader than it is. You have your own pants limitations, since if pants are too wide, the fullness can collapse around your hips and maybe even your thighs. Some skirt and dress styles offer more curve than your narrow hips can fill, and big bulky tops and jackets make you look like a boulder on top.

Just like you can't spot-reduce, you can't spot-gain either. Balancing this body feature, like all the others, is a matter of choosing the right clothing to create the womanly curves you desire, and with the following strategies, you will learn how.

There are three CASE strategies for narrow hips: Angle, Shape, and Shorten.

angle

▶ Fuller skirts that angle outward create a fullness in contrast to the narrowness of your hips and make them look wider.

▶ Sleeveless tops, halter tops, and armholes that angle inward balance narrower hips. Wide necklines, off-the-shoulder styles, and broad shoulder lines that angle outward make hips look narrower than they already are.

shape

▶ Shape the area of your hip with hip-building components such as embroidery and patch pockets.

shorten

▶ Wherever you add a horizontal line on the body, you automatically shorten that area and therefore make it look wider. Skirts with horizontal stripes will widen your hip area, as will pockets that are placed horizontally on your hip area.

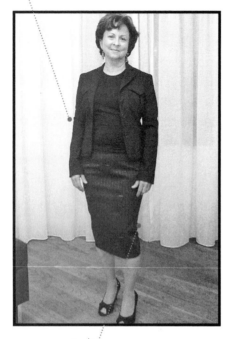

Narrow hips look narrower in a jacket that is less shaped.

Narrow hips look narrower in a pinstripe.

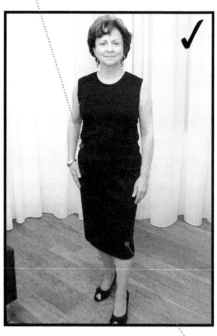

Narrow hips are widened with shaping in the waist.

Narrow hips are widened with a straight skirt.

Wherever vertical lines are placed on the body, they'll elongate and slim that area. If you have narrow hips, avoid making them look narrower by wearing vertical lines—such as pinstripes, for example. You can see in the photo on the right that our model's hips look wider than they do in the picture on the left. This is because the skirt she is wearing on the left has slimming pinstripes. If you have a choice between vertical stripes or no stripes, opt for no stripes at all.

Additionally, what makes her hips look narrow in the photo on the left is the shorter and boxier jacket she's wearing. Because this jacket creates a wider boxy shape on her upper body,

her hips look proportionately narrower. The picture on the right shows what happens when a top has more waist shape and sits closer to the hip area. The relationship between the top half and the lower half of her body is more of a match and makes her look less top heavy and more balanced than she looks in the photo on the left.

This does not mean that if you have narrow hips, you must swear off jackets for the rest of your life. When choosing a jacket, just make sure it has shape in the waist and is not too wide around your hips. Doing this will ensure more balance in your hip area.

In the photo on the left, because the shoulders of our model's jacket are so strong, her hips look narrower. In addition, because her narrow hips are emphasized with a slimmer skirt, she looks bigger on top.

Women with narrow hips look great in a fuller skirt because it adds fullness to an area that is naturally very slim. You can see in the photo on the right that because of the fullness created through the skirt, the model's hips look wider and her body looks more balanced. What is also causing her to look more balanced is the fact that her top has a softer shoulder line. This makes her shoulders look less broad and makes her hips look even wider

When choosing a skirt suit for narrow hips, choose a skirt with a bit of an A-line shape instead of a skirt that tapers so dramatically, and choose a jacket with a softer shoulder line that has a more rounded shape. Pegged, narrow skirts are not out of the question if you have narrow hips; just pay attention to the width of the shirt or jacket that you're wearing on top.

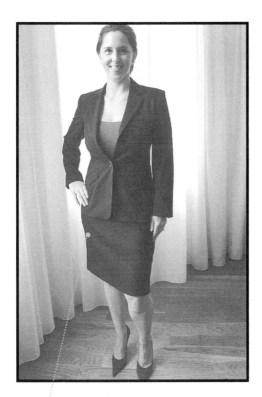

Narrow hips look narrower in a narrow skirt.

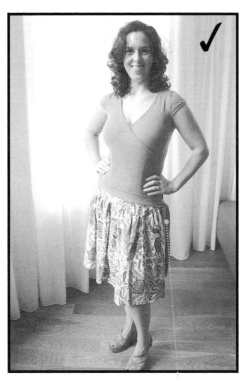

Narrow hips look wider in a fuller skirt.

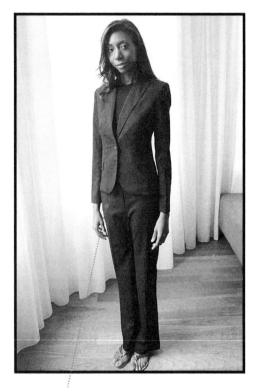

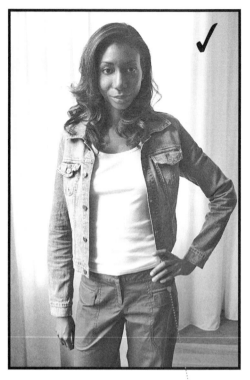

Narrow hips are narrowed with monochromatic colors.

Narrow hips are widened with patch pockets and horizontal lines.

In the photo on the left, our model's hips look longer and narrower because of the head-to-toe monochromatic coloring. Her body is elongated, making her look slimmer and her hips narrower.

Patch pockets placed in the hip area don't flatter many body types except for those with narrow hips. You can see in the picture on the right that by adding these patch pockets, our model's narrow hips look wider because of the widening horizontal lines created by the pockets and the extra bulk that patch pockets have.

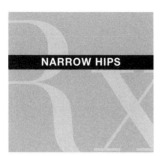

NARROW HIPS

- Wear fuller skirts.
- Build up the hips with details such as patch pockets in the hip area.
- Choose horizontal lines in the hip area.

If your hips are narrow . . .

- Look for pants made by European designers. European designers tend to cut much more narrowly in the hip and thigh areas of pants. American designers tend to make garments with a wider hip area because American women are traditionally known to have wider hips than their European counterparts.

- If your narrow hips can't fill out the hip shape of a skirt or pants, have your tailor reshape the hip area. This is an easy tailoring correction that isn't that expensive.

- Avoid creases on your pant legs if possible. Creases form vertical lines down the front of your pants, which will have an elongating effect. If you buy pants with creased legs, ask your dry cleaner not to press the creases when the pants are cleaned.

Big Butt

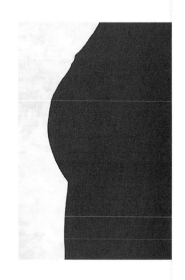

IF YOU HAD a nickel for every time you asked, "Does my butt look big?" you would be a millionaire by now (or at least a few thousand dollars richer). When you try on clothing, one of the first things you do is crane your neck around to see just how big your butt looks, and you are angry that you weren't more specific when you wished for dimples on your cheeks.

Whether or not you consider your big butt to be a round luscious peach or a flabby extension of your body that should have its own area code, the shape, size, and fullness of your behind are riddled with their own dressing challenges. As you slip your rounder, fuller butt into a pair of pants, excess fabric often gapes around your proportionately smaller waist, causing discomfort and offering an unwelcome peep show directly down to your underwear. You would rather stick pins in your eyes than take a peek at what your butt looks like in a bathing suit under the glaring fluorescent lights of a dressing room.

Even if the songs that celebrate a big butt make your bootie shake to the rhythm, they will never compensate for the feeling that your butt is some stranger lurking close behind you, one you'll never break free of. However, with the strategies presented below, you finally will.

All four CASE strategies are used for a large butt: Counterbalance, Angle, Shape, and Elongate.

counterbalance

▶ Counterbalance the fullness of a larger butt with fit-and-flare skirts and boot-cut pants. The fullness found at the hems of these styles balances the fullness of the butt and minimizes its size while giving it a flattering shape.

angle

▶ Angled or diagonal lines placed anywhere on the body have a slimming effect. A larger backside is slimmed with angled or diagonal lines such as stripes, seams, or diagonally placed pockets.

shape

▶ Big, fluid, shapeless skirts and pants will emphasize the size of a larger butt. Shape your rear with more structured skirts made of fabric with more substance and shape.

elongate

▶ When you elongate an area, you also slim it. Vertical lines placed anywhere on the body slims that area, making pinstripes

and any vertical seams placed over the derriere a slimming and balancing feature.

▶ Longer jackets that cover up the butt not only camouflage it but elongate the area, making a larger behind appear slimmer. Just make sure that the jacket has slimming shape in the waist.

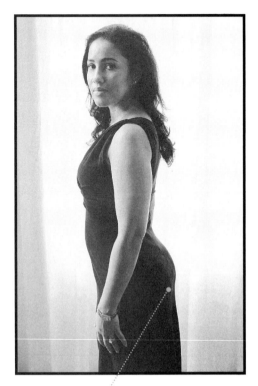

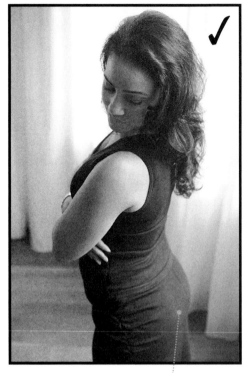

A big butt looks wider and wobblier in a skirt lacking shape and structure.

A big butt is contoured and shaped in a skirt with shape and structure.

In the picture on the left, the fabric of our model's skirt is not very substantial and is therefore not able to contain the shape of her butt. You can also see that the shape of the skirt does not shape the contour of her rear, and the skirt stands away from her body, creating a more triangular shape instead of a more natural rounded shape.

In the picture on the right, the skirt has shape and structure, which gives our model's butt shape and contour. The fabric of this skirt is more substantial and can contain the natural shape of her butt in a flattering way, therefore giving it a more rounded and balanced shape.

It is common for women to hide under skirts that have no shape or that stand away from their butt in an effort to conceal what they don't want to show. The truth is that when you choose a skirt without shape and contour, your butt looks bigger because of the way the skirt stands away from the body. In addition, if a skirt does not hug the natural curves of the butt, it is left on its own to move around in undesirable ways.

In the photo on the left, our model is fighting her own natural shape and, as a result, looks bigger, boxier, and wider. Because the shirt sits loosely at her waist and has no shape, she is bypassing the narrowness of her waist, which makes her whole body look as wide and full as her butt. Her stiff miniskirt isn't working with her own natural curves, and because it is sitting away from her own curviness, her butt looks boxy and square-shaped. The shortness of the miniskirt makes her butt look squatter; therefore, her butt looks wider and bigger.

In the photo on the right, our model is wearing an outfit that sits close to the shape of her butt and balances her natural curves. First, choosing a top that has shape in the waist, in particular the back of her waist, gives her butt a contoured and rounded shape that looks natural. Second, not only does the fit-and-flare style of the skirt shape and contour her natural shape, but the fullness at the hem counterbalances the size of her butt and makes it appear more balanced. Finally, because she is wearing a skirt that is knee-length, it elongates and slims out the fullness of her butt. Yes, you can tell that she has a fuller butt, but in this outfit, it is showcased in a positive way that balances her natural curves.

Instead of trying to cover up your butt with shapeless styles that you think will give the impression that you don't have a butt, go with the flow and embrace the natural curve of your body.

A big butt looks bigger in a shirt without shape.

A big butt looks balanced in a shaped top.

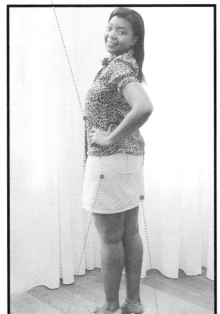

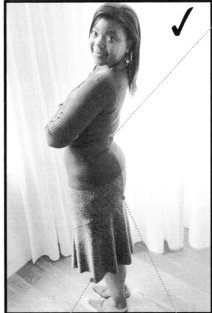

A big butt looks boxy and square in a stiff skirt.

A big butt looks squat and wide in a miniskirt.

A big butt looks balanced in a longer shaped skirt.

A big butt looks balanced in a fit-and-flare skirt.

Diagnosis and Prescription

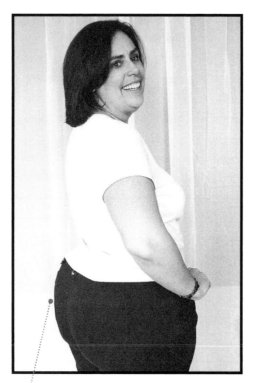

A big butt is enhanced with patch pockets and no vertical stripes.

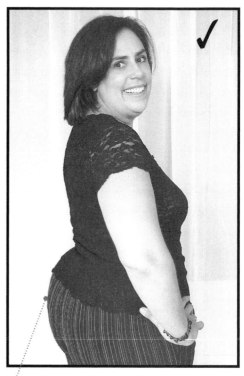

A big butt is minimized and balanced with vertical stripes.

Vertical lines have a slimming effect. In the picture on the left, our model's butt looks fuller and wider with no slimming vertical stripes on the pants. In addition, the patch pockets placed on her butt create a horizontal line across it, and horizontal lines placed anywhere on the body have a widening effect. Had these pockets been placed in more of a diagonal direction, they would have been more slimming because angled or diagonal lines have a slimming effect wherever they are placed on the body.

You can see that the vertical pinstripes in the pants on the right slim the shape of our model's butt. What is great about vertical lines placed over the butt area is that they not only have a minimizing effect in shaping but drastically narrow the width of the butt. Women who have large butts are usually more concerned with narrowing the width of their butt than embracing the natural curved shape that their fuller butt has. Vertical lines will certainly have a narrowing effect.

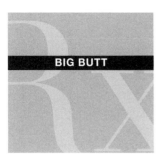

BIG BUTT

- Choose styles that shape your butt.
- Wear fit-and-flare skirts and boot-cut pants.
- Use angles and vertical lines to slim the butt.

If you have a big butt . . .

▪ Be careful about the types of back pockets you choose for your jeans and pants. Diagonally placed pockets will be more slimming as will back pockets that are larger in size. Smaller back pockets will look teeny in relation to the largeness of your butt and make your butt look even bigger.

▪ Avoid elastic waists in the back of your pants and skirts, especially in softer, drapier fabrics. With all that loosely gathered drapey fabric, the size of your butt will just be enhanced.

▪ Expect that you will most likely have to take your pants and skirts in at the back waist to compensate for the difference between the size of your butt and the size of your waist. This is an easy tailoring correction that can even be done on jeans.

Flat Butt

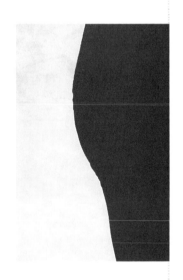

HAVE YOU EVER been asked if you mistakenly left your butt at home? Do you put on a pair of pants or a skirt and, when you turn around, notice that the clothing just hangs off your backside? If you can relate to any of this, then you are all too familiar with the struggle that comes with having a flatter butt.

Sure, there are tons of exercises you can do that claim to beef up your butt, as well as padding you can wear to give the illusion that you have more going on back there than you really do—some women even get surgical butt implants. However, you may not be that interested in walking lunge-style everywhere you go, and the last thing you would ever consider would be a plastic surgeon cutting into your derriere. So what is the alternative?

If you have less junk in your trunk than you would like, or if it appears that your trunk is completely empty, there is a way, with clothing, to create the impression of a fuller, rounder, and more ample butt.

The CASE strategies for a flat butt are Angle and Shape.

angle

- ▶ Angled stripes or seams on a skirt create the look of a shapely butt because angled lines provide more shape than vertical and horizontal lines, which have a flattening effect.
- ▶ A full skirt creates fullness and the look of a fuller butt.

shape

- ▶ Jackets with shape in the center back waist skim your waist, add some shape right above your butt, and give you more of a contoured shape, which makes your butt look rounder and fuller.
- ▶ A fit-and-flare skirt and boot-cut pants will add shape to your butt because of the contoured and rounded shape of these styles. Straight-leg pants and skirts that just lie flat on your butt emphasize the fact that there is a void where your butt should be.

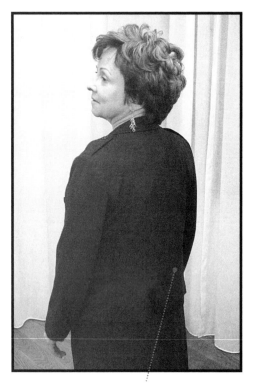

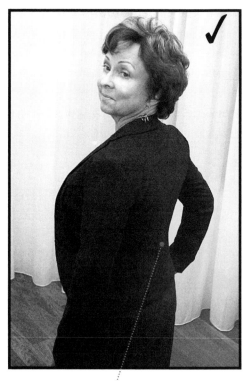

A flat butt looks flatter in a jacket with no shape in the back.

A flat butt looks fuller in a jacket with shape in the back.

It may be surprising to think that the fullness of your butt is dependent on how much shape there is in your tops and jackets, but looking at these two photos, you can see the difference a little shape makes.

In the photo on the left, there is no shape in the back of the jacket; there is just one straight line created from the lower part of the model's back to below her butt. It doesn't look like her butt can fill out the back of the skirt, and as a result, her butt looks flatter.

In the photo on the right, the shaping in the back waist of the jacket gives the model's lower back a rounded curve and some contour. She is shaped more like an *S* than an *I*.

In the photo on the left, even though our model's skirt is full, the fullness starts right below her butt. Therefore, this fullness emphasizes how flat her butt is. The horizontal lines running across her butt also make her look flat and wide because placing horizontal lines in an area that is already flat just makes the area look flatter.

The fullness of the skirt worn in the photo on the right gives the illusion that the model has more of a butt than she actually does. There is a secret to pulling this off: The skirt can't be stiff and hard because then it will just look like you can't fill it out. Instead, opt for a skirt that is full and has some structure as well as some movement, just like the one our model is wearing.

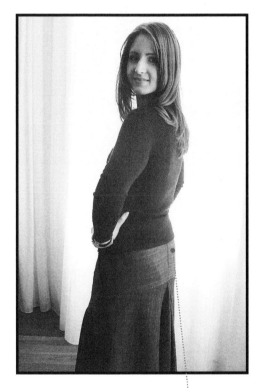

A flat butt looks flatter in a flat skirt.

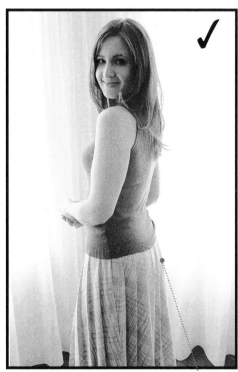

A flat butt looks fuller in a full skirt.

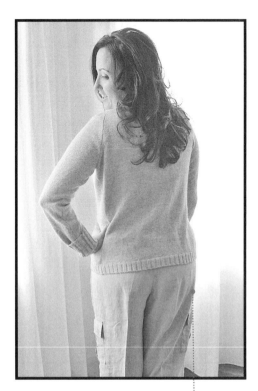

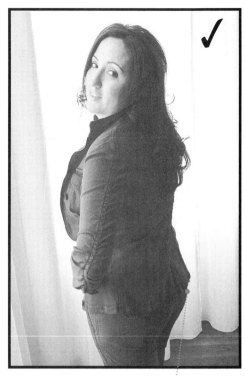

A flat butt looks flatter in a shapeless pant.

A flat butt looks fuller in a shaped pant.

I have stressed quite a bit that if you don't like what you have, don't hide it under bulky fabric— define the area with shape. In the photo on the left, the loose pants just hang off her butt, making it look as if she just can't fill them out. As a result, because her butt isn't shaped and contained, it looks wide and flat.

The picture on the right is a perfect example of shape defining in action. Our model may not have much of a butt; however, with enough shape in the pants, a rounder and fuller look is created. Her butt looks rounder and shapelier because her pants sit close to her body.

Also, the shape of the jacket in the photo on the right enables the model to create the look of

a rounder butt. The shapeless sweater in the photo on the left does nothing more than make her look flat.

Just as it is important to think about creating shape at your back waist to provide contour, the same is true for the back thigh area right below your butt. The more you shape it, the more shaped your butt will look. Does this mean that you should squeeze yourself into a pair of pants so that they look practically spray-painted on? Not at all. But if you look at the thigh area of our model in the photo on the right, you can see that her pants sit closer to the backs of her thighs than do the pants she is wearing in the photo on the left.

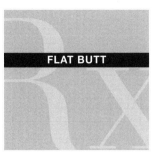

FLAT BUTT

- Use angled lines to make a butt look fuller.
- Choose a fuller skirt.
- Wear jackets with shape in the back.
- Wear fit-and-flare skirts and boot-leg pants to add contour.

If you have a flat butt . . .

▪ If you own jackets or button-down shirts that are straight in the back waist area, a very simple tailoring correction can make a huge difference. Just ask your tailor to take the jacket or shirt in at the back waist.

▪ Use three-dimensional elements such as patch pockets with flaps on your pants and skirts and back detailing such as bows on your butt area to create a fuller look.

Large Thighs

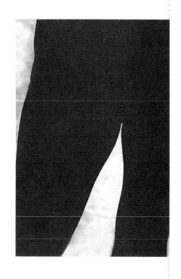

LARGE THIGHS ARE a body issue bestowed upon many women and, for you, an inescapable pain that makes finding the right pants impossible. Your large thighs may make you feel dumpy, bottom heavy, and possibly even sloppy.

Sure, we've heard that women who collect their weight in their thigh region have less of a risk for heart disease, and there are a number of good scientific reasons as to why women do, in fact, collect fat in their thighs. Science will also tell us that, even though you have done hundreds of leg lifts, the thigh area is one of the hardest spots for a woman to lose weight on her body. And let's not even discuss our *favorite* word—cellulite!

So what is the answer? The answer is in making the right clothing choices. The strategies in this section will help you flatter instead of emphasize your thighs, and teach you how to stop feeling as if your thighs were an annoying petulant child you have to drag around.

You will be pleased to know that one of the most common body concerns actually has the most solutions! Every CASE method can be utilized to tame large thighs.

counterbalance

- Tapered, narrow pant legs create a very unflattering "light bulb" shape; instead, counterbalance your thighs with a boot-cut pant style.
- Stiff A-line skirts can make you look squat and triangle-shaped; instead, counterbalance your thighs with a fit-and-flare skirt—a skirt that tapers at the knee and then flares out a bit at the hem.
- Wide necklines add much-needed width at your shoulder area and counterbalance a large thigh zone. Halter tops are not your friends.

angle

- Diagonal seaming or striping in a skirt or pants creates slimming angles in your thigh area and balances your thighs.
- Angled lines placed anywhere on the body have a slimming effect, so angled pockets on a skirt or pants will create an angled line that slims the area.

shape

- Fluid, drapey skirts in lightweight fabrics can cause your thighs to look sloppy and uncontained. Fuller thighs need to be shaped and contained with fabrics that are more substantial.

- Shapeless tops will only emphasize larger thighs. Defining your waist area through shaped tops, princess seams, and darts creates more of a balanced look for you and your thighs.

elongate

- Vertical lines elongate and slim an area. Vertical seams and pinstripes placed in the thigh area elongate and make them look slimmer.
- Monochromatic dressing elongates your body and makes your thighs look more balanced.
- Heels elongate your legs and have a slimming effect. Even if it is a small heel, they can offer a tremendous slimming benefit.
- Jackets that end right at the widest point of your thigh area call attention to your thighs; instead, choose longer jackets with shape that elongate and bypass your thigh area.
- Pants that fall straight from the widest point of the thigh will elongate and therefore slim the thigh area.
- Large thighs look better in skirts that taper more at the hem because they elongate and slim the area. Full skirts will shorten you and make your thighs look wider.

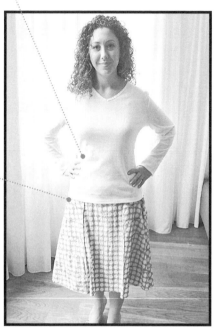

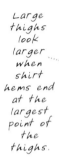

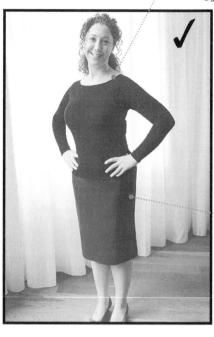

Large thighs look larger in shapeless tops.

Large thighs look slimmer with counterbalancing wider necklines.

Large thighs look larger when shirt hems end at the largest point of the thighs.

Large thighs look slimmer and more balanced in shaped and structured skirts.

I know that many women who have large thighs think an A-line skirt is the way to go, but as seen in the picture on the left, because the skirt is shaped like a triangle, the model looks like a triangle. In the photo on the right, a more tapered or pegged skirt makes her thighs look slimmer because of the elongating quality of the skirt. Areas of our body (like larger thighs) that can have an uncontained jiggle quality to them can be balanced or contained through clothing choices. The skirt in the photo on the right contains the model's thighs, giving them a slimmer appearance. The skirt on the left just leaves her thighs to run free.

Additionally, in the photo on the right, our model is wearing a monochromatic outfit that has an overall slimming effect on her body and makes her thighs look slimmer. The wider neckline that she is wearing counterbalances the fullness in her thighs, which minimizes the size of them. The shaping of the shirt in the photo on the right showcases her waist and not only minimizes the size of her thighs but makes her look slimmer overall. On the left, the shirt is less shaped. The top also ends at the widest point of her thighs, which calls attention to them and enhances their size.

Take notice where your eye focuses in these two photos. In the picture on the left, your eye goes straight to the thigh area, which is the area we are trying to balance, not emphasize or call attention to. In the picture on the right, your attention is at the shoulder area, which makes her look taller and leaner.

I will never forget a comment a fellow fashion designer shared with me: Pants that taper at the hem make women with large thighs look like lightbulbs or drumsticks. I keep this in mind whenever I work with clients who have larger thighs. If you have large thighs, you should never wear pants that taper or narrow at the hem. You can clearly see that our model's thighs in the photo on the left look wider as a result. If pants have a boot-cut hem, like the ones our model is wearing in the photo on the right, the width or fullness at the hem has a counterbalancing effect, making the width of the thigh look more balanced.

It is also important to point out how much more shape the jacket pictured on the right has in comparison to the jacket on the left. Most women who have large thighs usually have more of a defined waist in comparison to their thighs. Take advantage of the definition you have in your waist. You will look slimmer and taller, and your thighs will look more balanced. If you don't, you will look as wide as your thighs, as you can see in the photo on the left.

Also notice the difference in the shoes that our model is wearing in each photograph. In the picture on the left, because the toe of her shoe is more rounded, her legs look shorter and her thighs look wider and fuller. In the photo on the right, she is wearing a pointier shoe that matches closely to the color of her pant leg. Her legs look longer as a result, and whenever you elongate an area, you also slim it.

Large thighs look bigger in a jacket without much shape in the waist.

Large thighs are minimized with a shaped jacket.

Large thighs look bigger in pegged pants that taper at the hem.

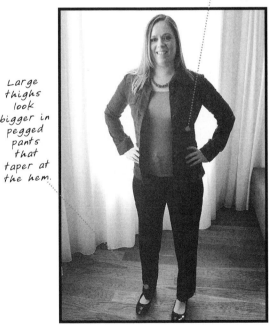

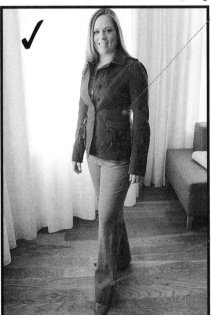

Large thighs are minimized with boot-cut pants.

Diagnosis and Prescription

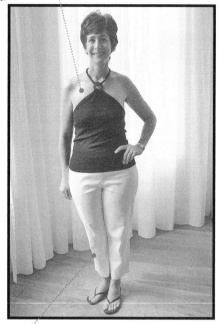

Full thighs look bigger in halter tops.

Full thighs look bigger in tapered pants.

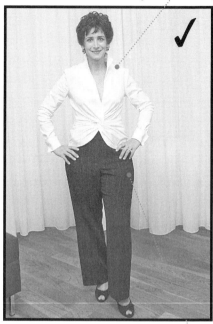

Full thighs look slimmer with a strong shoulder line.

Full thighs look slimmer in pants that fall straight from the widest point of the thigh.

In the photo on the left, the cropped pants shorten the leg, making the thighs look bigger and wider because horizontal lines placed anywhere on the body not only shorten an area but also widen it. The flat shoe has the same effect; even a slight heel would be better. Additionally, the halter top narrows her shoulders because of the way it angles inward, and this, with the effect of the tapered pants, emphasizes the width of the thighs.

Comparing this to the shot on the right, it is easy to see that there's a reason why every time we try pants on, we stand on our tiptoes. When we do this, we elongate the lower half of our body, therefore looking longer, taller, and slimmer. You can see this in the picture on the right. The more you elongate an area, the slimmer it looks. Because the pants hang straight from the widest part of her thigh, one straight line is created from thigh to hem, and she looks longer and therefore slimmer.

Due to the strength of the shoulder line in the photo on the right and how it counterbalances her larger thigh area, our attention and focus are drawn to the longer, thinner lines of her shoulder and face area, not her thighs.

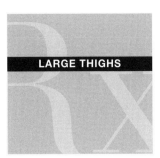

- Slim the thighs with boot-cut pants.
- Choose more structured, shaped skirts.
- Opt for wider necklines.
- Choose pants that hang straight from your thighs.

If you have large thighs . . .

- Stay away from pants with a tapered hem. If there are zippers at the hems of your pants, this means that the hem is so tapered and narrow that your foot can't fit through it unless you unzip the hem first. If you see zippers at the hem, run!

- Rein in your thighs using fabrics with structure; leave the lightweight fabrics at the store.

- If the outlines of your pocket bags show through your pants, have your tailor remove the bags and stitch the pockets shut.

- Bring the focus up toward your face with wider necklines and eye-catching elements such as earrings or necklaces.

- Big clunky boots with your pants tucked into them make your legs look squatty and your thighs appear wider because you are shortening the visual length of your leg, and when you shorten an area, you also widen it.

Short Legs

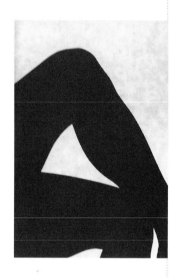

SURE, ITEMS THAT sit low to the ground have more stability. But when the items in question are your legs, you perpetually feel stumpy and find yourself wishing that everything in your wardrobe worked with a pair of tall platform boots, so that you don't look like you belong at the kiddy table.

For you, capri length means ankle length. You're putting your tailor's children through college with all the hemming you require, and wearing pantyhose means hiking the waistband somewhere up around your boobs. In addition, cargo pockets fall somewhere around your calves, full-length skirts and coats can make you look like you are standing in a hole, and a skirt with any type of a poof makes you look like one of those tacky doll covers used to hide an extra roll of toilet paper in the bathroom.

The good news is that you don't need to avoid wearing black-and-white color combinations for fear of being mistaken for a penguin. And your Achilles tendons can relax, as wearing four-inch heels isn't the only solution to making your legs look longer. With the strategies in this section, I am going to show you how to make your legs appear more greyhound than dachshund.

To lengthen short legs, the CASE method is to Elongate. Here is how to do it:

elongate

- Make sure your sleeves are not too long. The longer your sleeve, the shorter your legs look. Three-quarter-length sleeves are great if you have short legs, as they will make your legs look longer.
- Avoid big billowy sleeves because they have a widening and therefore shortening effect and will make your legs look short. Instead, choose slimmer and more tapered sleeves that sit closer to your arms.
- Shorter jackets are always a wiser choice for someone with short legs; long jackets just make your legs look shorter.
- Horizontal lines placed anywhere on the body shorten an area, so avoid cuffs on your pants, which will only shorten the look of your legs
- Narrower pants always look better because the closer they sit to your leg, the longer your legs look. Pants with a wider leg have a leg-shortening effect and will make you look like you are standing in a hole.
- Shoes that match your pants or your skin tone if you are wearing a skirt with bare legs will elongate the look of your legs.

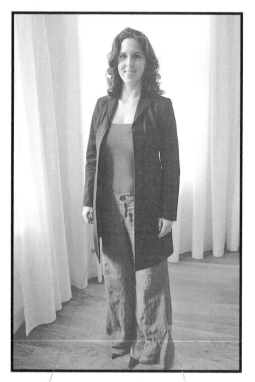

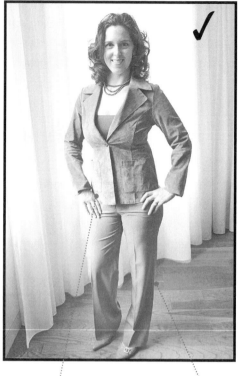

Short legs look shorter in a longer jacket.

Short legs look shorter in wide leg pants.

Short legs look longer in a shorter jacket.

Short legs look longer in a slimmer pant.

When you have short legs, the closer your pants sit to your legs, the longer you will look. This does not mean that your pants need to be tight or skin-fitting, or that you have to wear pants that taper at the hem. But if you look at the two photographs, you can see how the pants that are slimmer and fit closer to our model's legs make her legs look longer, while the wider pants in the photo on the left shorten the look of her legs. The fuller the pant leg, the shorter your legs will look.

The shorter jacket in the photo on the right makes the model's legs look longer. The shorter your jacket, the longer your legs will appear. In the photo on the left, you don't see much of her legs because a good part of them is getting cut off by the length of the longer jacket.

A long jacket and wide-leg pants are a lethal combination for someone who has short legs. If you want to wear a long jacket and you have short legs, wear it with either a short skirt or slimmer pants. If you want to wear pants with a wider leg, then wear a shorter, more shaped jacket or top. This will give your legs a fighting chance of looking a bit longer.

A full skirt is never a good idea when you have short legs. Full skirts, like full pants, create width on the body, and whenever you widen an area, you also shorten it. The more tapered skirt in the photo on the right sits closer to the model's body and is, therefore, more elongating because it is slimmer.

If you have short legs and want to wear a full skirt, try to find a skirt with the least amount of fullness as possible. You may want to look for something like the skirt on the right, a slimmer skirt with a small ruffle at the hem, that allows the model to have a soft, romantic look without

having to wear a full, feminine skirt that compromises the length of her legs.

Also notice the shoes in both photos. In the photo on the left, our model is wearing a flat shoe, and in the photo on the right, she is wearing a heeled shoe. This does not mean that if you have short legs, you can never wear flat shoes again. Heels will elongate your legs, but if you must choose a flat shoe, choose one that has a longer or pointier toe instead of a round toe, which cuts your foot off and makes your legs look even shorter. And opt for a shoe that matches the color of your skin, which will also make your legs appear longer.

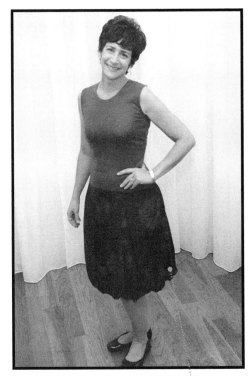

Short legs look shorter in fuller skirts.

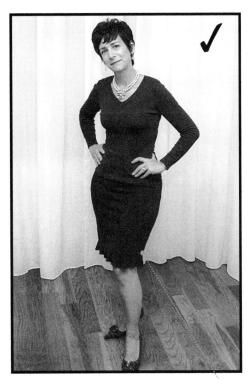

Short legs look longer in slimmer skirts.

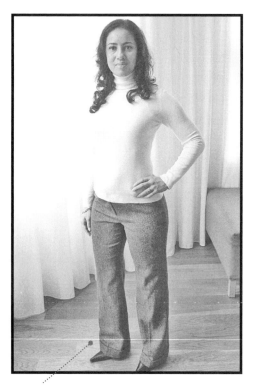

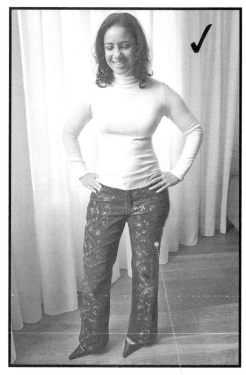

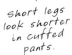
Short legs look shorter in cuffed pants.

Short legs look longer with vertically placed details.

In the photo on the left, the use of a horizontal line through a cuff shortens the appearance of our model's legs. Whenever a horizontal line is added to an area, it shortens that area, something you don't want when your legs are already short. Cuffs should be avoided if you have short legs.

Because of the vertically placed embroidery in the pants on the right, our model's legs look longer because vertical lines have an elongating effect. You can achieve this same effect with pinstripes, a crease, or a vertical seam running down the middle of the leg.

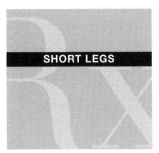

SHORT LEGS

- Hem the sleeves of your jackets and shirts if they are too long.
- Wear tapered sleeves.
- Don't wear cuffed pants.
- Avoid full pants and skirts.

If you have short legs . . .

- A creased leg on your pants will make your legs appear longer. If you buy pants without creased legs, creases are simple to add.

- Wear a shoe that matches either the color of your leg if you have bare skin showing, or the color of the pants or stockings you have on. By creating an uninterrupted monochromatic look from leg to toe, your legs will look longer.

- Avoid shoes that have horizontal straps across your instep; horizontal lines shorten, and straps will shorten the visual length of your legs.

Long Legs

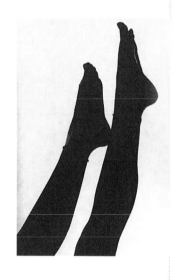

LONG LEGS: MEN like them, women want them, the Rockettes are famous for them. So what's the problem? Well, just because long legs look good doesn't mean that they don't come with their own share of issues, issues that go beyond there never being quite enough legroom anywhere you go. Having long legs can create plenty of clothing problems, many of which are all too common for you.

This may be a scenario you are familiar with: Excited by the possibility of an inseam being long enough for your legs, you grab a pair of pants from the rack with a tag marked *long inseam* and rush into a dressing room to try them on. While pulling on these pants in anticipation of finding a pair that isn't flood length, you find yourself remembering all the clothing hassles you have had to endure because of long legs. For fear of shrinkage, not one of your pants has ever seen the inside of a dryer, and you rarely wear heels with them. As you zip up the fly and inspect the hem, you let out a sigh of disappointment. Even these pants with the so-called long inseam aren't quite long enough for you. Frustrated, you get dressed again, leave the dressing room, and take a trip over to the shoe department to see if there are any ballerina flats on sale.

Long legs aren't only attached to women who look like they could play for the WNBA: You can be average to petite in height and have legs that are proportionately longer than the rest of your body. Whatever the case, you know you wouldn't trade or get rid of your long legs, but at the very least, you would like to know how to make them look more proportional to the rest of your body. With the CASE method, you will learn how.

To make your long legs look more balanced, the CASE strategy to use is Shorten.

shorten

- ▶ Fuller pants create width and therefore widen your legs, making them look shorter.
- ▶ Three-quarter sleeves and cropped pants make your legs look longer; either avoid them or avoid wearing both at the same time.
- ▶ Cuffs on your pants make your legs appear shorter; the deeper the cuff, the shorter your legs will look.
- ▶ Longer jackets shorten the look of your legs.
- ▶ Fuller, wider sleeves make your legs look shorter. Therefore, choose a fuller sleeve over a slim tapered one; a bell sleeve, which is a sleeve that flares out at the hem, will have the same effect.

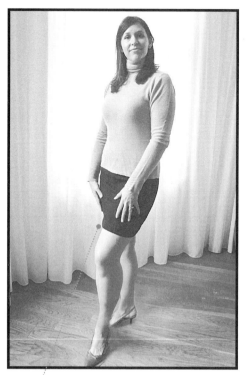

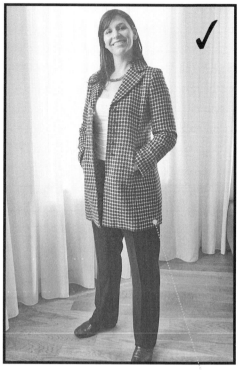

Long legs look
longer in a
shorter skirt.

Long legs are
shortened by a
longer jacket.

Short skirts just emphasize the length of the legs, as seen here in the photo on the left. What makes them look longer is the fact that her shoes match her leg color. If she wanted her legs to look shorter in this skirt, a darker contrasting shoe would have been a better choice.

The longer jacket worn by our model in the photo on the right cuts off the visual length of her legs and makes them look shorter. Women with long legs, especially tall women with long legs, look great in longer, shaped jackets. Also, the white top and black pants divide up the area between her torso and her legs and make her legs look shorter.

In the photo on the left, the model's legs seem to go on for miles. This model isn't tall at five-three, but she does have legs that are proportionately longer than the rest of her body. Without a cuff to stop the eye from seeing length, her legs look longer. In addition, because her top and bottom are the same color, her legs look even longer than they naturally are. The pointy toe of the shoe elongates the leg, and because the shoes match her pants and top, one continuous line from head to toe is created, making her legs look even longer.

It is hard for a woman who has very long legs to find a pair of pants that have a cuff. Most women with long legs use the excess cuff fabric to gain more length. Because of the cuffs in the pants in the photo on the right, her legs look shorter. Additionally, because her pants are a different color than her top, the horizontal line created where her top ends and the pants begin also makes her legs look shorter. Her darker-colored shoes also chop the length of her leg, making them look shorter.

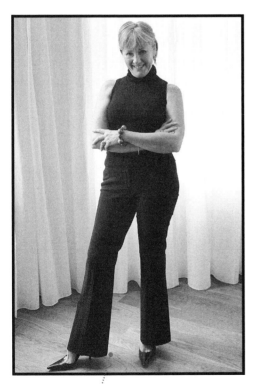

Long legs are elongated without a cuff.

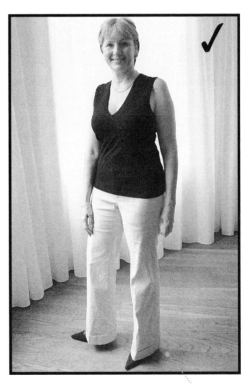

Long legs are shortened with a cuff.

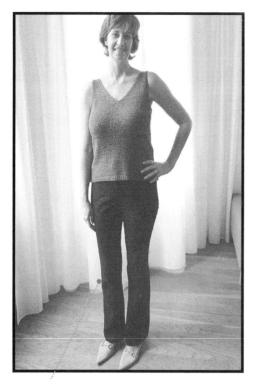

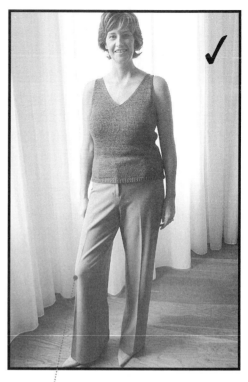

Long legs
look longer in
slim pants.

Long legs
look shorter in
wider-leg pants.

Clothing that sits close to the body also elongates it. You can see in the photo on the left that, because these pants fit closer to our model's legs, her legs look longer. If your legs are long and you want to wear slim pants, don't wear a shoe that matches the color of your pants; instead, choose a contrasting shoe color, which will have a leg-shortening effect.

Wherever you add fullness to an area of the body, you also shorten that area, and the full legs of the pants that our model is wearing in the photo on the right make her actual legs look shorter. Pants with a very full leg always work best on a woman who has long legs because she can spare the length that is lost when a wider leg pant is worn.

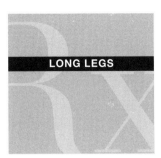

LONG LEGS

- Wear fuller pants and skirts.
- Avoid three-quarter sleeves.
- Wear pants with cuffs.
- Wear longer jackets.
- Choose fuller sleeves, which shorten the legs.

If you have long legs . . .

- Round-toed shoes shorten your legs; pointy-toed shoes elongate them.

- Avoid monochromatic looks or outfits that are all one shade if you want to shorten the look of your legs.

- It can be very challenging to find pants that are long enough for women who have very long legs. Few retailers can even meet the inseam demands of these women. Many retailers carry their longer-inseam pants online only, not in the store. It may be annoying that you can't walk into a store and leave immediately with a pair of pants long enough for you; however, an ounce of prevention is worth a pound of cure, and knowing ahead of time if you can get long-inseam pants at a store will save you the frustration of wasting time. Call ahead to make sure that the retailer carries long-inseam pants, or be sure to leave enough time to order online instead.

Large Calves
and Ankles

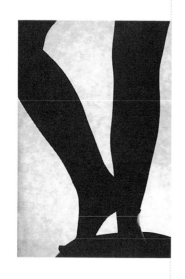

IF THERE IS one area that you and your large calves have the biggest issue with, it is shoe shopping—particularly shopping for boots. Does this situation sound familiar? While trying on a new pair of boots, you find that your excitement quickly wanes as you start stuffing your calves into the narrow boot while slowly, inch by inch, easing the zipper up your leg. Being very careful not to break the zipper, you notice that the skin on your index finger is starting to get raw from the effort and that beads of sweat are dripping from your forehead. Stopping to catch your breath before continuing on, you begin to wish there were a private place you could go and continue the struggle, as the public forum of the shoe store can be very humiliating.

Feeling defeated, you either give up mid-zip or, if you are really ambitious and up for the challenge, with enough sweat and sheer determination, you get the zipper completely up your calf. You notice, however, that just because you got the boot on does not mean that it looks particularly good. The leather of the boot surrounding your calf is stretched within an inch of its life, and you decide that the look just isn't working. As you unzip the boots, the sight of your calves expanding back to their normal size reminds you of raw Pillsbury biscuit dough swelling after the canister has been popped open. It is then that you decide that you can never wear boots, because all it takes is one humiliating experience to never try again.

Large calves don't discriminate. Your weight, body proportions, or size has no bearing on whether or not you have large calves and ankles, and there isn't much in the way of surgery or other drastic measures that can be done to eliminate this problem. Therefore, instead of begrudgingly accepting this feature and being fearful of being called out as the woman with the cankles, you can learn how to choose the right clothing to balance this figure feature. You can create a slimming effect, and you'll even find that with a few tips and tricks, you can actually wear tall boots. So let's explore the one strategy specifically made for you.

When you elongate an area of the body, it gets slimmer, so the CASE method for large calves and ankles is to Elongate. Here's how:

Elongate

- ▶ Vertical seams have a slimming effect, and when placed on boots, they elongate and slim out the width of the calf and ankle area.
- ▶ Skirts that end at the widest point of your calf widen the look of them. Instead, choose skirts that end at the narrowest part of your calf, which will elongate and slim the area.
- ▶ When wearing a skirt, choose a shoe that matches your skin tone or hosiery if wearing colored stockings or tights, as opposed to a shoe that is in contrast. When your shoes match your skin tone or stockings, your legs get elongated and your calves and ankles look slimmer.
- ▶ Avoid ankle straps on your shoes at all times. Ankle straps shorten the length of your calves, and when you shorten an area, you also widen it; therefore, your ankles and calves will look wide and thick in ankle straps.

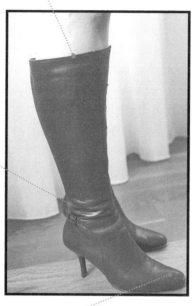

Large calves and ankles look larger when the boots and legs are two different colors.

Large calves and ankles look larger with horizontal lines on boots.

Large calves and ankles look larger in rounder-toed shoes.

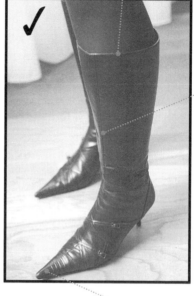

Large calves and ankles look slimmer when the boots and legs are all one color.

Large calves and ankles look slimmer in a boot with vertical lines.

Large calves and ankles look slimmer in pointy-toed shoes.

Few women with large calves could even imagine fitting them into a pair of tall boots, but being someone with large calves, I know from firsthand experience that it can be done (I'll share how later in this section). While you would probably be happy to get any boot to fit over your calves and ankles, there are some boots that are better suited for you than others.

Horizontal lines placed anywhere on the body enhance and widen that area. In the photo on the left, because our model isn't wearing stockings that match her boots, the horizontal line created where the boot ends and her leg begins makes her calf and ankle look bigger. In addition,

the horizontal line created by the buckle of the boot makes her ankle look wider.

A boot with a pointy toe will elongate the look of your leg and therefore make your calf and ankle area look slimmer, because the more you elongate an area, the slimmer it looks. In the photo on the right, there is also a vertical line going down the front of the boot, which makes the calf look narrower. In addition, when wearing a boot, choose a stocking color that matches the boot, which will create a monochromatic look. Because of this monochromatic dressing, the leg gets elongated and ultimately looks slimmer.

It is very common to grab a pair of black shoes to wear no matter what your outfit. However, if you have large calves and ankles, you should consider otherwise. The photos below show the same skirt with different shoes. In the photo on the left, our model's calves look heavy and her ankles wide. The reason is that the black shoe is so much darker than her skin tone that it breaks up the leg, shortens it, and makes it look larger.

The photo on the right shows why you should never underestimate the power of shoes that match your skin tone. They create an elongated seamless look in the calves and ankles, making them look slimmer.

If you still aren't sold on the power of skin-tone shoes and you must have black ones, then wear the finest black shoes you can find. The chunkier the black shoe, the chunkier your calves and ankles are going to look.

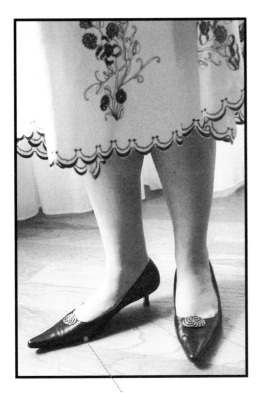

Calves and ankles look heavier in a shoe that is darker than the skin tone.

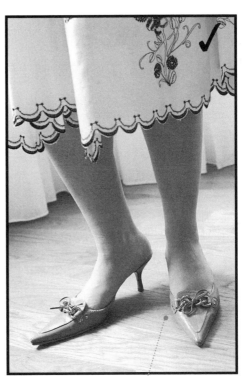

Calves and ankles look slimmer in a shoe that matches the skin tone.

Diagnosis and Prescription   131

Large calves and ankles look larger when a skirt ends at the widest point of the calves.

Large calves and ankles look slimmer in a skirt that ends at the narrower part of the calves.

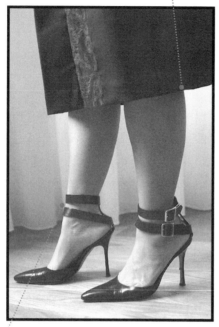

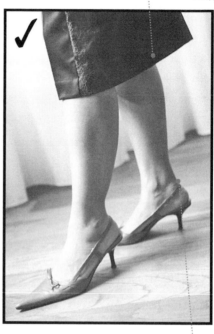

Large calves and ankles look larger in ankle straps.

Large calves and ankles look slimmer when ankle straps are avoided.

It may be hard to believe, but this is the exact same model in both photos. In the photo on the left, because our model's skirt ends at the widest point of her calves, they look much heavier. The strap around the ankle cuts the length of her legs off even more, and as a result, her ankles and calves look thicker.

In the picture on the right, the length of the skirt is slightly shorter and ends at the narrower part of her calf. Her calf looks slimmer because the slimmer part of her calves are exposed. Additionally, because the shoes don't strap

around the ankle, her foot is elongated, which has a slimming effect and makes her ankles and calves look leaner.

An improper skirt length can be easily corrected. Always hem skirts to hit the same point that the skirt on the left hits: the slimmest part of your calf. I also can't overemphasize how important it is to avoid ankle straps if you have large calves and ankles. If you love ankle-strap shoes, then choose a color that is close to your skin tone, or wear them only with pants so that the straps are hidden.

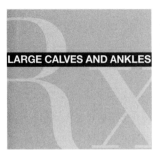

LARGE CALVES AND ANKLES

- Choose boots with vertical seams to slim calves.
- Be sure your hemlines hit the narrowest part of your calves.
- Match your shoes to your skin or stocking color.
- Don't wear ankle straps.

If you have large calves and ankles . . .

▦ Can't get a pair of boots over your calves? Have them stretched out. Many shoemakers will stretch the calf portion of a pair of boots. I had a pair that needed to be stretched so much that they had to be kept on the stretcher for a week. In the end, the boot was stretched two inches wider to fit over my calves.

▦ Leather does stretch over time, so if boots are a bit snug in the shoe store, most should stretch out and fit over your calves after a few wears.

▦ Many tall boots have elastic in the calf part of the boot. Keep your eye out for these styles, which will stretch with you and fit over your calves.

Thin Calves and Ankles

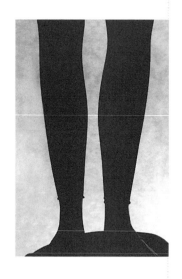

YOU HAVE CHICKEN legs that would have made Frank Perdue drool with envy. However, impressing Mr. Perdue isn't high on your priority list. What is a priority for you (and your thin calves and ankles) is looking like you're not supported solely by two toothpicks.

Because of your thin calves and ankles, you often find yourself puncturing an additional hole in an ankle strap so it can fit tight enough around your ankle. Tall boots are so roomy that they swim around your calves, making you look like a swashbuckling pirate. And with the excess bulk that pools around your ankles when you wear stockings or tights, you feel as attractive as an elephant.

It isn't that you wish for thick, bulky calves in exchange for the lithe ones you have, but a little curve would be nice. Lucky for you, there are ways to make your calves and ankles look fuller and curvier, and with the CASE strategy for this problem, you'll learn how.

Whenever you want to widen an area, shorten it. This is your CASE method for adding shape to thin calves.

shorten

▶ Ankle straps shorten the leg and therefore make the calf and ankle area look wider.

▶ A narrower pant leg that sits close to your leg creates less space between your pants and your calves and ankles, which makes them look wider.

▶ Shoes that don't match your skin tone shorten the look of your legs, making your ankles and calves look wider.

▶ A flatter shoe shortens the leg, making the ankle and calf area appear fuller.

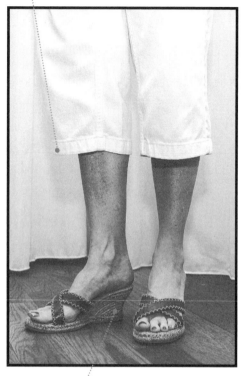

Thin calves and ankles look thinner in wide-leg pants.

Thin calves and ankles look thinner in heeled shoes.

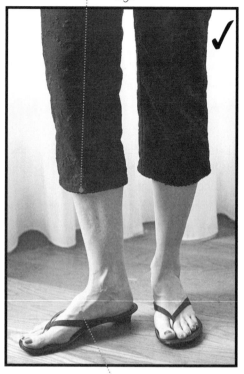

Thin calves and ankles look bigger in pants that sit close to the leg.

Thin calves and ankles look bigger in flatter shoes.

The wider the legs of your pants, the skinnier your legs are going to look. In the photo on the left, with such a wide leg on the pants, the thinness of the ankles and calves is emphasized because there is so much width around them. Also, a higher heel elongates the leg, and when you elongate an area, you also make it look slimmer.

In the photo on the right, with the pants hugging the legs closely, the calves and ankles look fuller because there isn't a lot of space between the model's calves and the pant legs. The fact that she is wearing a flatter shoe also makes her ankles and calves look wider because the leg is shortened.

This rule applies particularly to cropped pants, where your ankles and calves are on display for all to see. Choosing a hem that sits closer to the calf is the better choice if you have thin calves and ankles.

It is important to point out here that the model in these photos is a plus-size woman who has very thin ankles and calves in proportion to her thighs. In the photo on the left, our model is wearing a shoe without any ankle straps, and because there are no horizontal lines to break up the slimness of her leg, it looks thinner and less curved and shaped.

In the photo on the right, her ankles look fuller. The ankle strap she is wearing places a horizontal line over a thinner part of her leg, and wherever you place a horizontal line, that area appears fuller than it actually is. The horizontal line also gives her calf more shape and curviness, which is a common desire with most thin-calved gals.

Thin calves and ankles look thinner and straighter in a shoe without ankle straps.

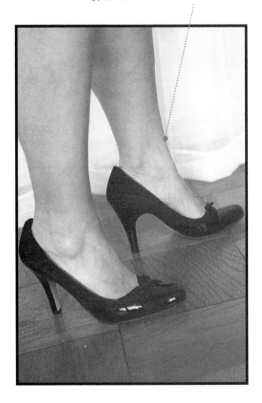

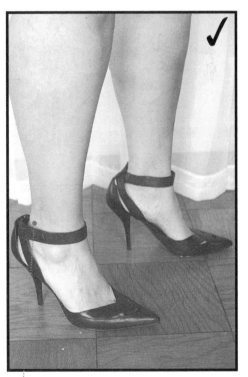

Thin calves and ankles look curvier and fuller in ankle-strap shoes.

Diagnosis and Prescription

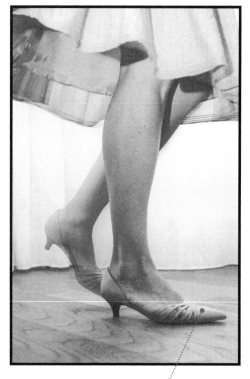

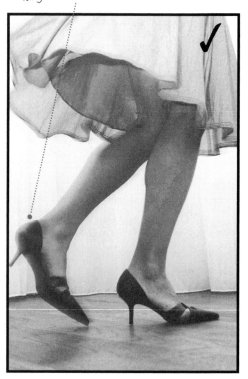

Thin calves and ankles look thinner in lighter-colored shoes.

I have shown repeatedly that whenever you shorten an area of the body, that area also gets wider in appearance. In the picture on the left, the matching color of the skin and shoes elongates the legs, and by elongating the legs, our model's calves and ankles look even slimmer than they already are.

In the picture on the right, you can see how the darker shoes, in such contrast to the color of her skin, shorten her legs and makes her calves and ankles look wider.

If you have thin calves and ankles, I am not encouraging you to wear black shoes with white stockings just because this creates a contrast— that look is not very fresh. But if your bare legs are showing and you want your ankles and calves to look a bit heavier, then wear a shoe that is darker than your skin tone.

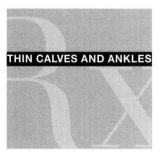

- Wear ankle straps.
- Wear narrower hems on your pants.
- Choose shoe colors that contrast with your skin tone.
- Choose flatter shoes over heels.

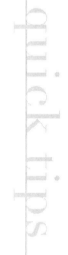

If you have thin ankles and calves . . .

- Just as boots can be stretched to fit over large calves, boots can be made narrower in the calf area by your shoemaker.

- Boots with stretch in the calf area should fit snugly over it.

- Not only do ankle straps make your ankles look wider, but so do Mary Jane–style shoes that have a strap over your instep. The horizontal line from the strap shortens your leg and makes your ankles and calves look wider.

- Opt for more round-toed shoes over pointy-toed shoes; the roundness of the toe has a shortening effect and will make your calves and ankles appear fuller.

Wide Feet

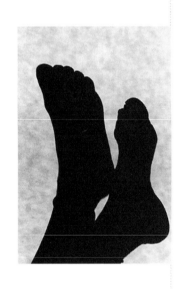

IF YOU HAVE wide feet, then you've probably experienced the disappointment of learning that the shoe you want isn't available in the wide width or, worse, that the store you're in doesn't carry wide shoes at all. You find yourself skulking around the shoe displays, wondering if you should just force your feet into a pair of narrow, pointy-toed shoes, then you swear you can actually hear your toes shrieking in horror at the very idea. As the number of possibilities dwindles rapidly, you try to concoct creative solutions to the challenge of how you can leave the store with a pair of shoes that fit.

You consider buying shoes in a half size larger, hoping that the extra length may give you some extra width. Sometimes this works; other times you end up walking right out of those larger shoes once they stretch from wear. Since pointy-toed shoes are out, you consider open-toed styles, but they make your toes look like a package of Vienna sausages, and only you can understand how embarrassing it is when the sides of your unsightly feet spill over the edges of a pretty, strappy sandal.

With the often scant shoe offerings in wide styles and those creative measures you've been forced to take to cover up your feet, it is easy to feel like an outcast who has been destined to a life of sensible shoes in ugly styles. You aren't asking for the world—you simply want attractive shoes that don't make you a permanent fixture in your podiatrist's waiting room. It may have worked for Wilma Flintstone to walk around in a fabulous outfit sans shoes, but for you it is not an option. While I may not be able to persuade shoe departments to offer more wide styles, there are definite strategies you can employ to make your feet appear narrower than they are. In this section, I am going to show you how.

Wide feet benefit from the following CASE strategies: Counterbalance, Angle, and Elongate.

counterbalance

▷ When a wide foot is counterbalanced with a wider heel, the foot looks balanced and thinner. A tiny heel only emphasizes that a foot is wide.

angle

▷ Angled or diagonal lines are lines that slim. Shoes with angled details narrow and taper the look of a wide foot.

elongate

▷ Vertical seams in a shoe elongate and narrow the foot.

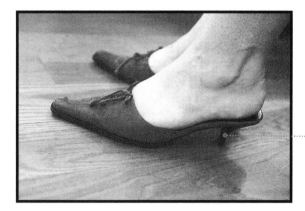

Wide feet look wider in a small heel.

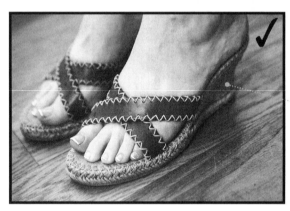

wide feet look narrower in a heel that is more substantial.

Wide feet need to have enough width support or they will look wider than they already are. Looking at our model's feet in a pair of shoes with a delicate heel in the photo on the top, her feet spill over the sides of the shoe and the smallness of the heel makes her feet look wider than they already are.

In the photo on the bottom, the thickness of the heel matches the width and thickness of our model's foot, thereby making her foot look more balanced and narrower. In addition, because angled lines have a slimming effect, the diagonal lines of the straps make her foot look narrower.

Horizontal lines placed anywhere on the body have a widening effect. In the photo on the top, the wide horizontal created by the strap going over the instep widens the look of the feet. While it is important to choose a shoe that can contain the physical width of your foot, it is also important not to choose a shoe that is too wide in appearance because it will just make the foot look massively wide, as this shoe is doing here.

Because diagonal lines have a slimming effect, the diagonal lines in the shoe pictured on the bottom help create the look of a narrower foot.

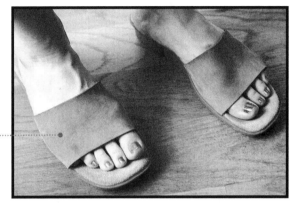

Wide feet look wider with horizontal lines.

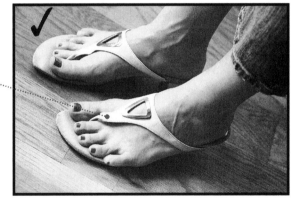

Wide feet are narrowed with diagonal lines.

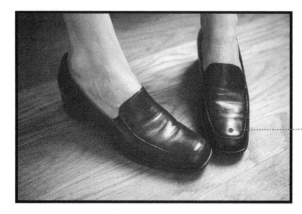

Wide feet look wider in square-toed shoes.

Wide feet look narrower in pointy-toed shoes.

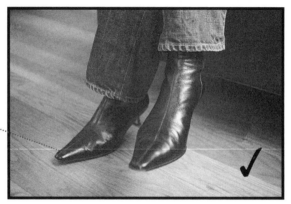

A shoe that cuts across the instep horizontally, pictured on the top, always makes a foot look wider than it already is because horizontal lines widen an area. A better idea is to choose shoes without such a severe horizontal line across the instep. The square toe is also making the foot look wider because it is shortened with such a square shape. A more tapered toe would be a better choice. A solution to this shoe style would be choosing a sock or stocking color that matches the shoe. Because the model's bare skin is showing, a contrast is created between it and the shoe. A matching sock or stocking creates a seamless monochromatic color, making the horizontal line on her instep less obvious.

Anytime you add a vertical line to a shoe or boot, the foot looks narrower because vertical lines have a slimming effect. As you can see, the vertical line in these boots, pictured on the bottom, elongate the foot and therefore make the foot look slimmer. Also the tapered toe of the boot elongates, making our model's wider foot look slimmer as well.

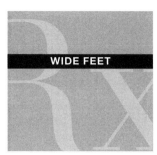

WIDE FEET

- Wear shoes with a thicker heel.
- Use angles and vertical lines to narrow wide feet.

If you have wide feet . . .

- Some women have wide feet but the backs of their feet are narrow, limiting them to shoes that have a supportive strap over the instep. A solution to this problem is to have a shoemaker use a heated tool to narrow the backs of your wider-width shoes.

- Choose shoes that match your skin tone or the color of the stocking you are wearing. By creating a monochromatic or singular shade from leg to foot, the foot looks narrower.

- Avoid shoes with any three-dimensional detailing on them, such as buttons and bows. Your foot is wide enough, so you don't need any additional bulk on your shoes.

quick tips

Narrow Feet

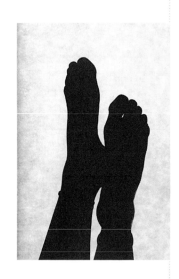

EXCITED TO TRY on a new pair of shoes, you look down to admire them, only to be quickly disappointed. The shoe is so much wider than your foot that it looks like it could devour your foot with one quick bite. You can probably stick a finger or two between your foot and the side of the shoe, and you wonder which would be worse: wandering the world barefoot for the rest of your life or wearing uncomfortably wide shoes that don't fit. After years of wearing too wide shoes, you are beginning to think the former.

To find shoes that snugly conform to your foot, you've tried sizing down but find yourself burdened with blisters and permanently curved toes. You play blister round-robin, wearing a pair of shoes that look great yet hurt and don't fit, and then rotate to another pair that hurts in a different place on your foot, leaving you with several blisters at a time, all in different stages of healing. There are serious shoe limitations when you have narrow feet, including wearing shoes that you are clearly settling for. You can't just pop into the store on a whim to find that perfect shade of green that matches your new designer suit because you feel relegated to the few shoe stores that actually carry narrow styles. Often frustrated, you wish you didn't have to wear shoes, which could easily become a reality because, with your narrow feet, you could walk right out of a pair.

Sure, the upside to narrow feet is that they look fabulous in shoes, and if you could just stand around looking pretty, everything would be fine. But heaven forbid you also have to walk. With the CASE strategies, you won't find a magic wand that will make your foot immediately widen. But you will learn how you can make your slender foot look wider and more proportionately balanced with the rest of your body.

Your two CASE strategies are Counterbalance and Shorten.

counterbalance

▸ A chunkier heel will make your foot look even narrower. Instead, opt for a finer and narrower heel whenever possible.

shorten

▸ Horizontal lines have a shortening and widening effect. Therefore, when they are placed across your instep, your foot will look wider.

▸ Vertical lines have a slimming effect, and will therefore only make your foot look longer when on a pair of your shoes. Avoid them whenever possible.

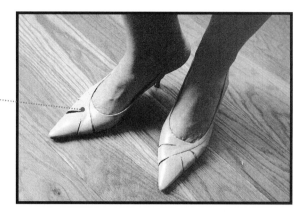

Narrow feet look narrower with angled or diagonal lines across the instep.

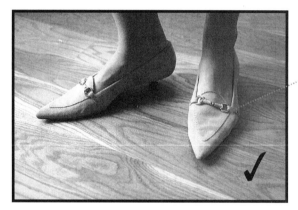

Narrow feet look wider with a horizontal line across the instep.

In the photo on the top, the angled pattern in the shoe makes our model's foot look longer and narrower—exactly what you want to avoid. An angled or diagonal line will make an area look slimmer.

Anytime you place a horizontal line where an area is narrow, that area automatically looks wider. You can see in the photo on the bottom that the horizontal line on the instep of the shoe widens the model's feet.

If you put a chunky shoe or heel on someone who has a very narrow foot, that width will only make her foot look even narrower. In the photo on the top, with such a clunky shoe and heavier heel, our model's foot can't fill out the shoe; therefore, her foot looks much narrower. Even the horizontal line across her foot doesn't do enough to make her foot look any wider. A better solution would be to choose a shoe in a color that is darker than her skin tone, because the darkness would shorten the look of her foot and make it look wider.

In the photo on the bottom, you can see that the finer shoe and slimmer heel match the fineness of our model's foot, and as a result, her foot looks wider.

Narrow feet look narrower in a chunkier shoe and heavier heel.

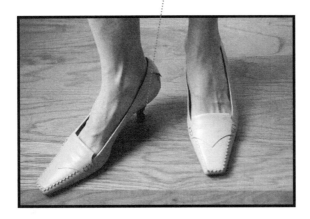

Narrow feet look wider in a finer shoe and heel.

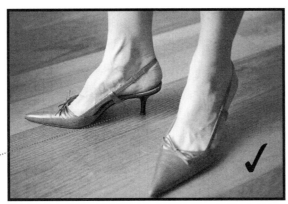

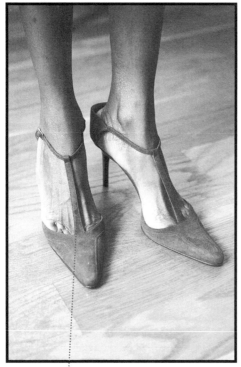

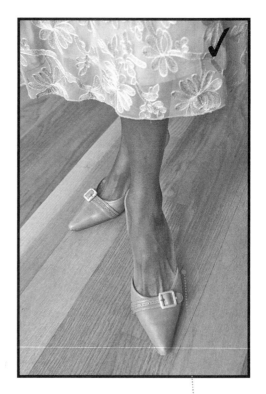

Narrow feet look narrower with vertical lines in the instep.

Narrow feet look wider without vertical lines.

When your foot is narrow, the last thing you want to do is make it look narrower through adding a vertical line right down the middle of it. Vertical lines slim any part of the body, and in the photo on the left, you can see just how much her foot is slimmed by the T-strap of the shoe. Instead of a T-strap, a basic ankle strap without the vertical strap down the middle of her foot would have made her foot look much wider.

In the picture on the right, you can see how the absence of a vertical line in the instep makes the model's foot look wider. It is clear that sometimes when we do nothing to an area, it looks wider than if we do something to it.

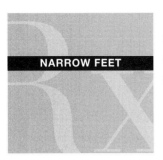

NARROW FEET

- Wear finer, thinner heels.
- Select shoes with horizontal lines to widen the foot.
- Avoid vertical and angled lines on your shoes.

If you have narrow feet . . .

- Choosing shoes with bows, buckles, or any other three-dimensional detail will increase the visual width of your foot.

- Try using padded inserts placed right under the ball of your foot for better fit when shoes are too wide.

- Choose shoes that are in contrast to the color of your skin tone; the contrast creates an appearance of width and fullness in your feet.

- Rounder, squarer, and less pointy toes shorten the look of your feet and make them look wider.

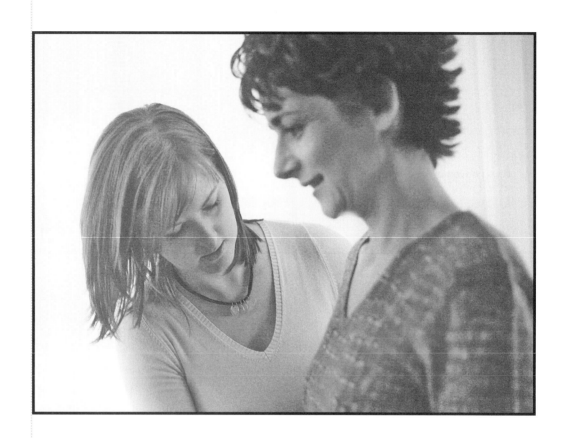

PART II

Balance and Harmony

YOU ARE THE most important part of the dressing equation, so while it's important to choose the right clothing for your body, all the strategies I shared in Part I can quickly become a wash if you're not the shining center of attention in what you wear. That perfectly fitting jacket may make you feel washed out, or that dress may be the perfect shape for your figure, but the print seems all wrong. There is a big difference between getting the compliment "That's a really nice skirt" and hearing "You look great!" I'm guessing that if you're like me, you'd rather receive the second compliment—one that recognizes you and not just a skirt! In this part, I'm going to share the extra strategies that will take you from simply wearing great, well-fitting clothes (the first compliment) to actually looking great (the second one!).

It has been said that being stylish means to stand out and fit in at the same time, and I couldn't agree more. When you wear clothes, there should be a seamless synergy between you and what you put on your body. Take a moment to recall a person who tried really hard to *appear* stylish. How did she look? As if she tried too hard perhaps? Or maybe you didn't notice her—instead, all you saw was her clothing, and she was in the background somewhere. Take a moment now to think of someone who *is* stylish. Everything in her wardrobe seems so compatible with her that her style is seamless; her clothing choices are so perfect that when she's wearing them, they're secondary to her.

Don't get me wrong, I (obviously) love fashion. This isn't an antifashion statement, nor am I going to give you strict rules that will have you swearing off certain fashion choices. Instead, you'll learn to make informed decisions that will ultimately help you wear your clothing versus your clothing wearing you. You can have the best of both worlds. You can be incredibly stylish *and* have your clothing be about you at the same time—you don't have to compromise.

In this section, we'll step away from the body and talk about your face. By exploring your facial characteristics, you'll learn how to create a look that makes *you* stand out and shine. Some of these tips and strategies are inspired by things I learned during my image-consulting training as well as what I taught my clients and the dramatic effects they've had.

In addition to teaching you how to wear your clothing versus your clothing wearing you, this part will enable you to make quicker, smarter decisions when shopping. Let's face it, who has time to roam around clothing stores without a sense of purpose and then come home either empty-handed or with choices that weren't made with confidence? Imagine if you could scan a rack of clothing and just grab an item knowing you are choosing the thing that is ultimately a compliment. What would it be like if you didn't even have to pick through piece by piece, glazed over and clueless? What would it be like if racks of clothing could be eliminated at first glance? After reading Part II, you'll find out.

Intensity

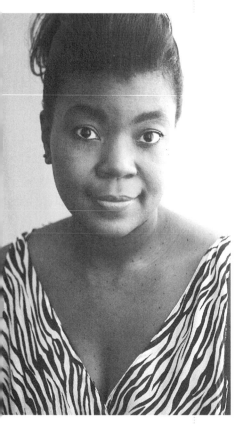

HAVE YOU EVER put on an outfit, only to feel like you have suddenly become invisible? Have certain prints either drowned you or made you look washed out but you aren't sure why? In this part, you'll find out why these scenarios may occur and what you can do to avoid them.

This picture explains it perfectly. Our model is wearing a black-and-white patterned top. We could probably all agree that the print she is wearing is pretty bold.

The black-and-white color combination is what makes the print appear bold, and because of this boldness, it overpowers our model. Do you notice that your eyes keep focusing on the print the model is wearing and not the model herself? The reason? A little something called intensity level.

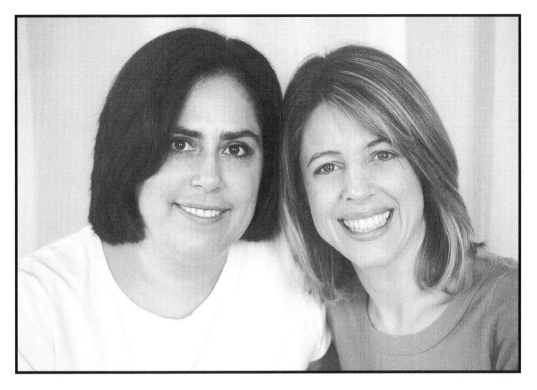

What is intensity level?

Intensity level is the boldness or softness of one's personal coloring. Intensity level varies from person to person and can be bold, soft, or somewhere in between those two extremes. Your intensity level is determined by the relationship of contrast that is created between the hair, skin, and eyes. Let's take a look at some examples to help you better understand this key dressing point.

Comparing the two extremes

Taking a glance at the two women in the photo, it is obvious that they look different. Our model on the right has a softness to her color-

ing. You may notice a similarity in shade among her hair, skin, and eyes, and because of this similarity, there is an evenness to her coloring. She has what would be referred to as a soft intensity level.

Our model on the left has fair skin just like our model on the right. However, her hair and eyes are much darker in comparison to her skin tone. There isn't one similar shade among her hair, skin, and eyes; in fact, the coloring of her hair and eyes is in complete opposition to that of her skin. Because of this opposition, a bolder level of intensity is created in her own personal coloring.

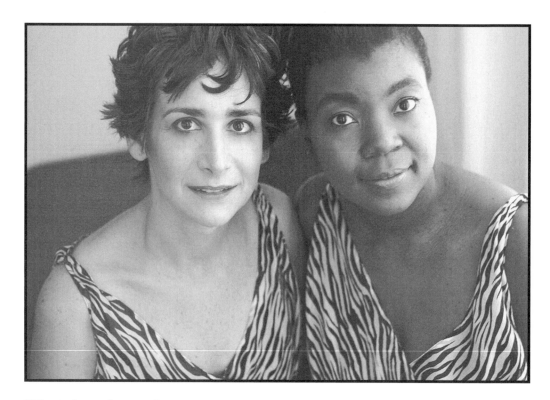

What does intensity have to do with it?

When choosing the level of intensity in your clothing, it is important to consider your own personal intensity. Let's take a look at this photo for clearer explanation.

Look at our first model again in that same black-and-white top. Now that you are starting to understand intensity level, you can tell that she has a soft level of intensity in her personal coloring because of the similarity of coloring among her hair, skin, and eyes. In this photo, she is sitting with another model wearing the same black-and-white top. Because the model on the left has hair and eyes that are much darker than her fair skin is, she has a much higher intensity

of coloring. Can you see that the personal intensity level of our model on the left matches the boldness of the black-and-white pattern that she is wearing? Intensity of the print plus the intensity of her bold coloring equals a perfect match between coloring and clothing.

Black and white isn't always right!

While it is a common color combination for many women to wear, few women can actually wear black and white! Why? When you combine a dark color like black with a light color like white, what gets created is a very bold and optic combination that, unless your personal intensity level can match it, will drown you out.

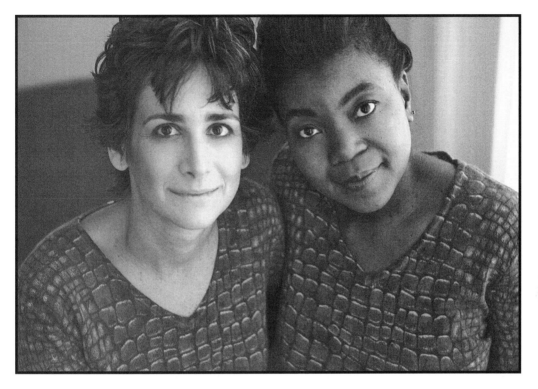

Let's now look at a picture of the same models both wearing a different top. This time the intensity of the color combination of the top they are wearing is much softer and not nearly as bold as the black-and-white combination in the first top. Can you see how a soft print works well on a person with a lower level of intensity and washes out a person whose coloring is much bolder?

You will always look best when the level of intensity in your clothing matches the level of intensity in your coloring.

Take a look at the following examples.

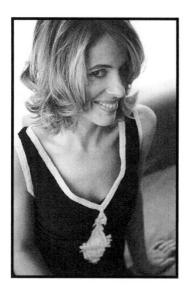

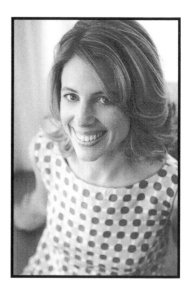

The black-and-white combination of this dress steals the show and is much bolder than our model's personal intensity.

The print of this dress is a perfect match for our model's coloring; you notice the dress and the model equally.

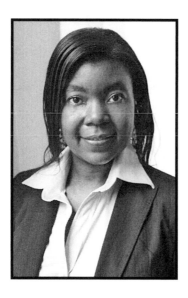

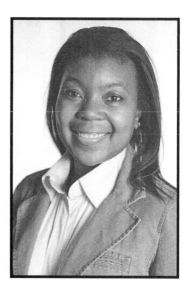

A darker jacket over a lighter shirt creates a bold color combination and drowns our low-intensity model out.

If we simply lighten up the color of the jacket, the combination becomes a better match to her own personal coloring.

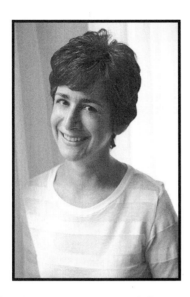

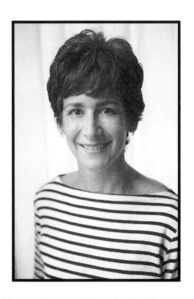

A soft stripe isn't intense enough for our model and washes her out.

A bolder stripe matches the boldness of our model's coloring.

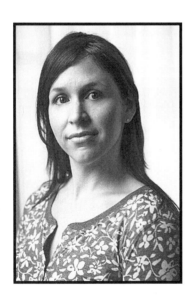

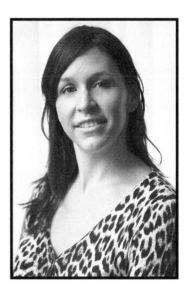

The softness of this print just can't rise to the occasion and match the bold intensity of our model's coloring.

The boldness of the print is a perfect match for our model's bold personal intensity level.

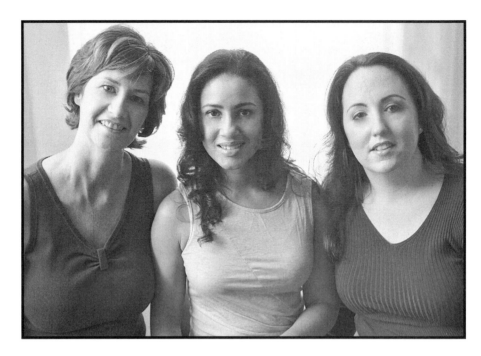

The sliding scale of intensity

Take a look at your own level of intensity: Is it as bold or soft as the models we just looked at? What if your intensity level isn't bold or soft? Looking at your own coloring, you may notice that you seem to fall somewhere in between the two. This isn't uncommon; in fact, most people fall somewhere on a sliding scale between the two opposites of bold or soft.

Let's explore this a bit further. At first glance, the models pictured in this photo all seem to have different coloring. However, even though they look different, they all have one thing in common: Their coloring isn't as bold as the bolder-intensity models we looked at earlier, and it isn't as soft as the softer-intensity models either. Medium intensity allows for a much broader coloring range, and each of these

women falls at a different place on the scale between soft and bold.

The model on the left has a softness of coloring but not nearly as soft as someone who would be considered to have a lower intensity of coloring; therefore, she would fall on the lower side of the medium-intensity scale because of the very slight amount of boldness in her coloring. The model in the middle has very dark hair and eyes, but her skin isn't as fair as the models we looked at who have a bolder intensity level, which is why she has more of a medium intensity level. Finally, the model on the right is the boldest of the three. Her skin is fair and her eyes and hair are dark, which creates some boldness, but her eyes and hair aren't as dark as the models we previously defined as having a bold intensity.

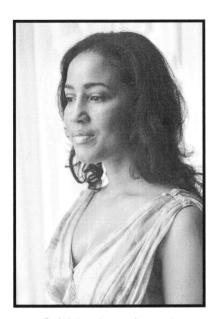

Soft intensity washes out.

Color combinations for the medium intensity level

So what does a person who has a medium level of intensity wear? Remember, you always look best when the level of intensity in your clothing is a perfect match to the level of intensity in your own coloring.

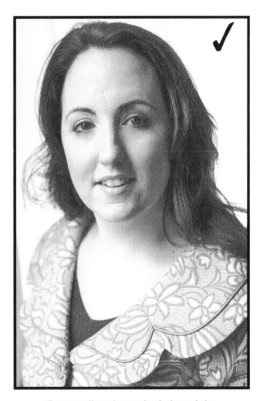

But medium intensity is just right.

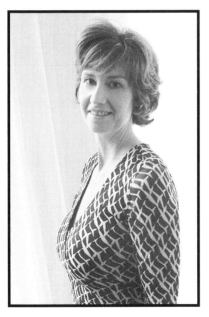

Bold intensity drowns out.

Here are some more examples of the best choices for someone who has a medium amount of intensity in her personal coloring.

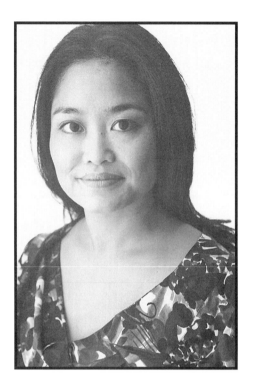 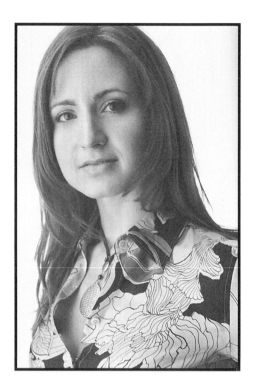

The model on the left may have very dark eyes and hair, but her skin tone gives her a medium level of intensity. That is why this print works so well on her. If this print were just black and white, it would be too optic and bold, but the gray softens the print and works with her coloring.

The model on the right has very fair skin and her eyes are very deep, but because her hair isn't as dark as someone with a bolder level of intensity, she falls into the medium level. A bold print like black and white would drown her out, so the slight softness in this print works perfectly with her coloring.

Determining your own level of intensity

So what is your intensity level, and how do you determine it? If after looking at the photos of these models you are still having a hard time identifying your level, use the following scale to help you.

MY HAIR COLOR IS:	Light		Medium		Dark
MY EYE COLOR IS:	Light		Medium		Dark
MY SKIN COLOR IS:	Light		Medium		Dark

Place an X on the line between Light and Dark where you think the coloring of your features falls. The more similarity shared by all three features, the softer your intensity level; the greater the difference among the three features, the more bolder your intensity is.

Here's an example of a filled-out chart:

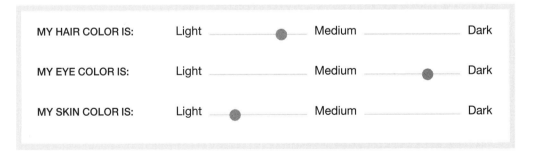

According to the chart, this person's hair color is between being light and medium, her eye color is between medium and dark, and her skin color is between light and medium. Because of this, her contrast would fall in the medium category.

Let's revisit some of the photos we looked at earlier to help you understand this even better.

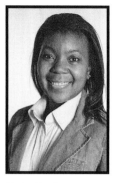
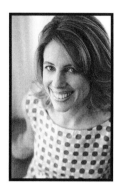
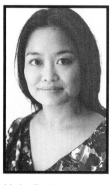
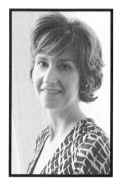

Hair: Dark
Eyes: Dark
Skin: Medium Dark
Intensity: Medium
       Soft

Hair: Light
Eyes: Light
Skin: Light
Intensity: Soft

Hair: Dark
Eyes: Dark
Skin: Medium
Intensity: Medium

Hair: Medium
Eyes: Medium Dark
Skin: Medium Light
Intensity: Medium
       Soft

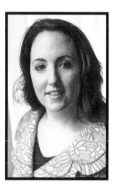
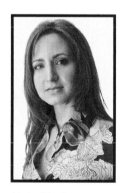
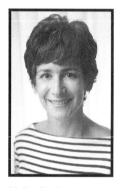

Hair: Medium Dark
Eyes: Medium
Skin: Light
Intensity: Medium
       Bold

Hair: Medium
Eyes: Dark
Skin: Light
Intensity: Medium
       Bold

Hair: Dark
Eyes: Dark
Skin: Light
Intensity: Bold

Final thoughts on intensity

If it's good enough for models, why isn't it good enough for me?

I'm sure that you've seen many advertisements of a low-intensity model wearing an outfit with a high-intensity print or pattern. This may make you wonder, If they do it in magazines, then how can it be a mistake? The truth is that it isn't a mistake for advertising, but that doesn't mean it's okay for you. Clothing ads are selling the clothing, not the model wearing it. Therefore, it would make sense that they would put an outfit with bold intensity on a model with soft intensity because the clothing stands out and the woman practically vanishes.

You aren't selling your clothing; you're selling yourself—and I have yet to meet a woman who wants her clothing to get more attention than she does.

Does intensity level change?

I have often been asked if intensity level can change, and the answer is yes. In the summertime many people tan, making their skin tone darker and their intensity level lower. Also, over time, dyed hair can lighten, altering your intensity level. Just because your intensity level changes with the seasons or the different phases of your hair coloring cycle doesn't mean that you have to have a completely different wardrobe to accommodate

each change. You may find that your summer wardrobe varies a bit from your winter wardrobe, or that you have a slightly different color combination with that fresh coat of hair color, but for the most part, even with these changes, your intensity level stays pretty much within a similar range—unless you go and do something drastic like completely change the color of your hair to a much darker or lighter shade!

Does this mean that I can never wear black and white again?

With all this newfound knowledge, it may seem that wearing black and white together is now reserved for the few out there who resemble Snow White. Can you only wear color combinations if they match the intensity level of your own personal coloring? Of course not. Remember, the information I am sharing with you throughout this book isn't about creating limitations in your wardrobe but about providing a way for you to make informed decisions. There are always days when it is more important that we get noticed over our wardrobe, whether you're giving a presentation, interviewing for a new job, or trying to stand out in a crowd. In these situations, when you want to be seen over your clothing, working with your intensity level is an asset. But if you are running errands, scrubbing your bathtub, or playing with your kids at the park, the fashion police certainly aren't going to arrest you for breaking any wardrobe laws.

Texture

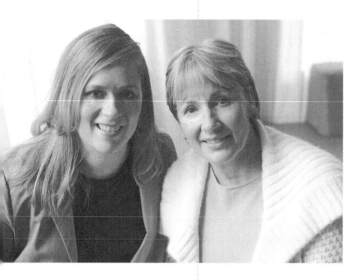

WHILE SHOPPING FOR clothes, you have probably noticed the vast array of fabrics with different looks and feels. Some fabrics have a lot of texture or surface interest, resembling those shag carpets from the seventies. Other fabrics have a smooth feeling to them and can be so shiny that we practically see our reflection when we look at them. Between these two extremes are an unlimited number of fabrics that feature different textures and looks.

Looking at the two models in this photo, you can see that they are wearing different amounts of texture in their clothing. Our model on the left is wearing a leather jacket that not only looks smooth but would feel smooth to the touch. Our model on the right is wearing a sweater that has a lot of surface interest, or texture.

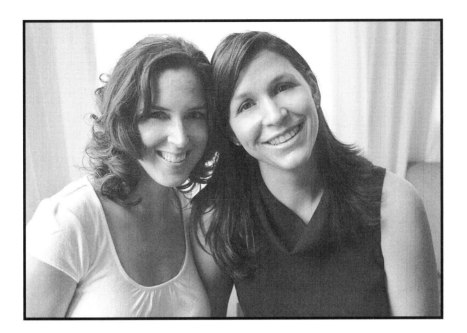

It is important to be aware of the different textures in the fabrics that make up clothing. Choosing clothing has just as much to do with fabric as it does with the shape and silhouette that you prefer. This section explores the texture in fabrics and how it enables you to wear your clothing versus your clothing wearing you.

The two models pictured here look very similar; their hair, skin, and eye color are practically the same. There is one big difference between these two models, however, and it has a dramatic effect on their clothing choices. One model has straight hair and the other model has curls. While you may not immediately think that this difference has any effect on clothing choices, it actually does. Because of her curly hair, the model on the left has a more textured appearance, while the model on the right, with her smoother hair, has a much smoother appearance.

The textural qualities of our appearance play a big part in how we can successfully choose the types of fabrics that are best for us to wear. Let's take a look at why.

A textural match

The more texture you have in the physical appearance of your hair, such as curls or waviness, and your skin, such as wrinkles or blemishes, the more texture you can successfully wear in your clothing. The reason is that the smoother your hair and skin appear, the better you will look in smoother, less textured fabrics because there will be a match between your facial appearance and your clothing. If you have smoother skin, the more overpowering a textured fabric will look on you. If you have more texture in your hair and skin, fabrics that are too shiny or flat, or without any texture, will just look flat on you and can even enhance the textural quality of your skin.

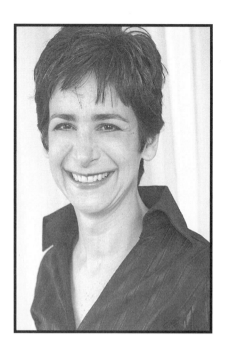

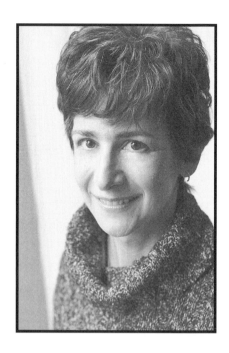

Better than Botox

Be it aging or skin imperfections, one of the best ways to camouflage any skin imperfection is to wear textured clothing. Textured skin is emphasized when fabric that is too smooth or shiny is worn, because the shinier fabric makes the texture of your skin appear more obvious. Many of us fear aging; however, few of us realize that our clothing choices can often counteract any anti-aging routines we rely on to look younger. Alternatively, however, the fountain of youth can often be found through our wardrobe choices. Who knew that bouclé could be as effective as Botox?

Let's take a look at some examples of the effect that texture in our clothing can have on our appearance.

The model pictured here has curly hair, and even though her skin is smooth, the amount of texture in her hair gives her overall appearance more of a textural quality. Looking at her in a top with some shine, you can see how she doesn't look completely balanced. Because her skin is smooth, she does have a bit more flexibility with wearing flatter fabrics than someone who has more texture to her skin. Therefore, this top still works on her. However, if our model had both textured skin and textured hair, this flatter and shinier top would be even less balanced, and if she had wrinkled skin, the shine would enhance her wrinkles.

By putting a sweater on her that has a lot of texture, there is a match created between what she is wearing and her face, and you notice her face instead of just the clothing. What she is wearing and her physical features become one, creating a unity and sense of balance between the two.

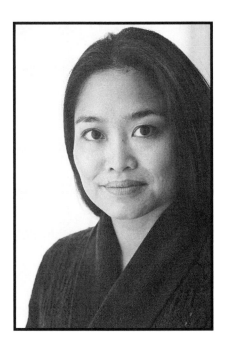 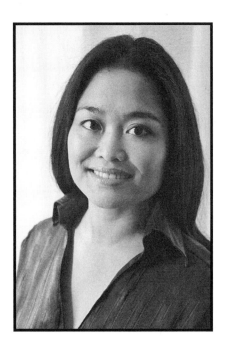

In the photo on the left, you can see how the smallest amount of texture on someone with very smooth hair and skin doesn't work as well as a top with less texture does. A better sweater choice for her would be a flatter knit with no surface interest or texture.

In the photo on the right, the model is in the same top that the previous model was wearing.

While the other model, with a more textured appearance, looked acceptable in the top with a bit of smooth shine, the model pictured here wears the top better simply because she has an overall smoothness to her appearance, and because there is a match between her appearance and her clothing, she has a more balanced overall look.

Here we have the same model in two very different tops. In the photo on the left, she is wearing a shirt that has a lot of texture, although she doesn't have a lot of texture in her hair and skin. As a result, the top is wearing her instead of her wearing the top.

In the top she is wearing on the right, the level of texture is smooth just like her hair and skin, and she gets to shine as much as the top does.

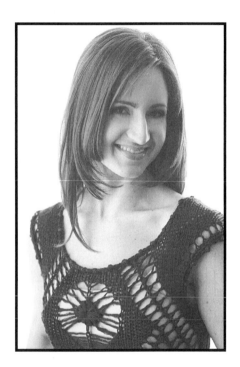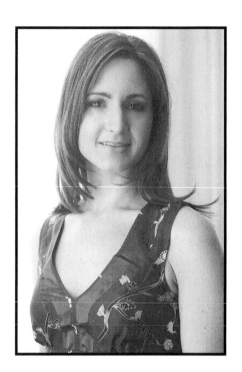

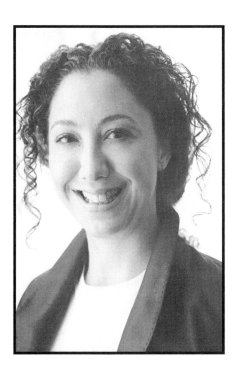 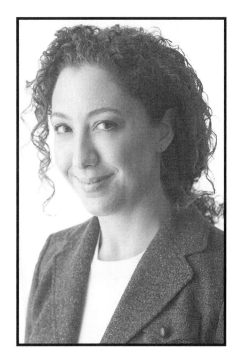

In the picture on the left, the sheen and flatness in the jacket the model is wearing aren't a match to all the texture she has in her hair. As a result, harmony isn't created between her and the jacket, and the jacket isn't nearly as flattering as the jacket with more texture.

While her skin is very smooth, the model has very curly hair, and as a result, she looks much better in texture. As you can see in the picture on the right, even the small amount of texture found in the jacket makes for a better match for the textural qualities of her appearance. Your focus goes right to her face instead of getting caught up solely in what she is wearing.

So what is your texture level? Use the scale below to help you determine it:

MY HAIR'S TEXTURE IS:	Smooth	Medium	Textured
MY SKIN'S TEXTURE IS:	Smooth	Medium	Textured

Simply place an X where you feel the level of texture in your hair and skin falls. The more texture you have in your hair and skin, the more texture you can wear in your clothing, and vice versa. Here's an example of a completed chart:

MY HAIR'S TEXTURE IS:	Smooth	●	Medium	Textured
MY SKIN'S TEXTURE IS:	Smooth	Medium	●	Textured

In this chart, the Xs indicate that this person has textured skin, presumably because of blemishes, wrinkles, or other skin imperfections. She also has slightly textured hair. With regard to clothing, she would look best in more textured fabrics, as smoother, flatter, or shinier material would not balance her face, and her skin imperfections would also stand out more.

Here's another example of a completed chart:

MY HAIR'S TEXTURE IS:	Smooth ●	Medium	Textured
MY SKIN'S TEXTURE IS:	Smooth ●	Medium	Textured

In this case, the person's texture in both her hair and skin is very low; therefore, she should choose clothing that has a smoother, flatter appearance. Anything too textured would overpower her face and wear her instead of the other way around.

Final thoughts on texture

What if I have smooth skin but textured hair?

If your skin is smooth but your hair is textured, you really do have a lot of flexibility. You can wear smoother fabrics because of your smoother skin and can also wear textured fabrics because of your textured hair. When choosing smoother fabrics, opt for more of a matte quality than too much sheen, and try to keep a balance of both smooth and textured in your wardrobe.

What if I can't tell how much texture a surface has?

As I said earlier, there are varying amounts of texture out there. Fabrics don't have to just have sheen to be considered low texture. The less surface interest a fabric has, the less texture it has. When you aren't sure as to how much texture is in a garment, just close your eyes and run your hands over the fabric.

Keep in mind that not all textured fabrics are devoid of sheen. Velvet, for example, would be considered a textured fabric because there is a nap or raised quality to the fabric. However, most velvets also have a shiny quality to them, so if you do have more texture in your personal appearance, it is wise to leave velvets for the lower-textured gals.

This also does not mean that if you have a higher level of texture in your appearance you can never wear fabrics with sheen—such as satins—again. The best way to wear these fabrics is with some added surface interest, such as embroidery or pleats gathered in a way that creates texture. While suede may be better than leather for someone who has a lot of texture in her appearance, leather is also an option; if you wear animal skin, I suggest choosing a skin that has some textural quality to it instead of one that is very shiny.

And what about the basic fabrics that make up your pants, suits, and jackets? The texture rule still applies. If you have a smoother appearance, a flatter fabric without any surface interest would be a smart choice, but if you have texture in your appearance, all it takes is the smallest amount of a textural weave—a simple tweed, for example—to add some dimension to the fabric.

Movement

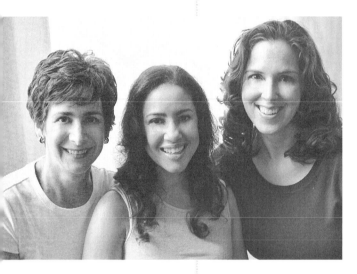

WHENEVER I START working with a client, I always ask her if she wears a lot of prints or patterns. Many clients tell me they don't. While I have always felt that the decision to include prints or patterns in one's wardrobe is one of personal preference rather than something a client must do in order to achieve a balanced wardrobe, I still ask them why this is the case. Many clients tell me that they would be very open to wearing prints but often feel confused by all the choices and what would be best for them. As a result, many women don't even bother buying prints and commit to a wardrobe full of solid colors.

Selecting prints is a very personal undertaking, and we often feel as if we are choosing wearable artwork. This is why style, tastes, and personality factor heavily when deciding what prints to wear. Using your own gut reaction and seeking out what attracts you visually can be a smart and effective way to look for prints. However, personal choice and instinct alone aren't always reliable, and that's why many women who go with their gut don't always make the right decisions. I have had clients with very bold personalities look foolish in ditzy, irreverent prints that don't speak to the aura of personal power they naturally give off, and I have also had very demure, soft-spoken clients who look overpowered by a print that gives off a lot of power and energy.

The missing element in finding the right prints is looking at the features of your own face. As I have said in preceding sections, the best way to get noticed in your clothing is for your clothing to support the features of your face. Therefore, the face is an important consideration when choosing the right prints.

Facial movement

Facial movement is the way the features of our face move. Features can move in ways that are soft and round or in ways that look sharp and angular. Let's take a look at the models pictured on the previous page to get a better idea of this concept.

The model on the left has features that are very geometric or linear. Her eyebrows are more horizontal than angled or curved; the shape of her eyes, even though they have a slight round-ness, has more of a linear quality; and even with a smile, her mouth moves very horizontally. The bridge of her nose is more defined than the tip, making her nose look very vertically shaped.

The model pictured in the middle has much rounder or curved features. Her eyebrows have a softer arch, her eyes are much rounder, she has rounder cheekbones, and her smile is much softer. The tip of her nose is more prominent than the bridge, making her nose softer looking. Unlike our first model, she has an overall softer and rounder look to her face.

The model pictured on the right has very diagonal or angled features. Her eyes have a diagonal shape and movement to them. Her eyebrows have more of an angled arch, the shape of her nose is more angled, and her smile has a very angled quality to it.

Just as our facial features all move in different ways, so do prints. Some prints are geometric and linear; others are soft, rounded, and fluid. Still others have a combination of harder lines with softer shapes. There are plenty of different print shapes and styles out there to choose from, which is why decision making often gets very confusing.

The best print styles for you would be ones that move in ways that match the way your own personal features move. If you have very rounded or soft features, then a very round and soft print would be the best choice for you. If your features are much more angular or geometric, then a print that is more angular and geometric would be a good choice.

Let's look at some examples.

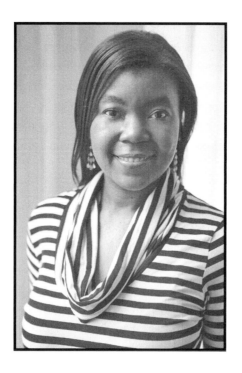 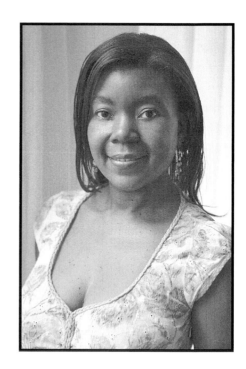

The model pictured here has features that are very soft and round. Her eyebrows, eyes, nose, cheeks, and mouth are all very round in appearance.

In the picture on the left, the horizontal stripes are very linear. Can you see how the model's face fights the harsh lines of this top? Instead of there being an overall balanced look between her face and what she is wearing, there is a struggle created between her face and her top.

As a result, you don't notice her as quickly because the top distracts you from seeing her.

The print she is wearing on the right is a much better choice for her because the print itself is also very round in appearance. The soft round-ness of the floral pattern matches the shape and movement of her softer, rounder features, and because a match is made, there is balance between her and her clothing. As a result, she is wearing her top instead of it wearing her.

This is the model I mentioned at the beginning of this chapter, the woman with very diagonal or angled features. In the top on the left, the round polka-dot style looks pretty, but it is hardly as workable as the argyle top she is wearing on the right. The movements of the dots are too soft and round for her more angled features, and there isn't as much synergy created between the model and what she is wearing. Because the shape of her eyes, eyebrows, nose, and mouth all move diagonally, she looks perfect in the argyle sweater, whose pattern has that same diagonal movement. A marriage is made between the face and what she is wearing, and with a look that is so seamless, she will get noticed.

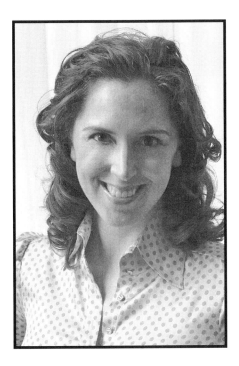 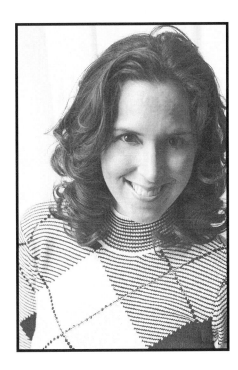

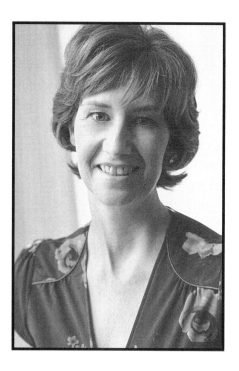 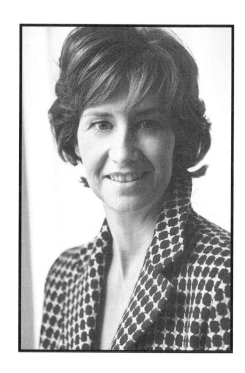

The model pictured here has more linear features. They don't angle or move diagonally, as the previous model's features did. Instead, this model's features move more horizontally and vertically. Her eyebrows are hardly arched and are much straighter. The shape of her eyes is more linear and less round, and her smile is much more horizontally shaped than the other models we looked at. In the photo on the left, such a round print looks too soft and round for her features. As a result, she doesn't look as pulled together as she does in the more geometric pattern seen on the right. A face with such linear, geometric movement looks great in prints and patterns that move more geometrically or in a linear fashion, as does the jacket she is wearing on the right. Because the linear movement of the jacket matches the linear quality of her features, the look between her face and what she is wearing is seamless.

Some people don't have features that are as singularly distinct as the models we have been talking about. Many times someone may have a combination of several feature movements, like being linear and round at the same time.

You can see in the two photos here that these two don't have features that move as obviously as our previous models. The model on the left has a softer, rounder shape to her eyes and nose, but the shape of her mouth is much more linear. Her eyebrows are more angled and arched.

Because of this true combination of angles and softness, the best print choices for her would be shapes that aren't too linear and geometric nor too round or soft, like the shirt she is wearing.

The model pictured on the right is also a combination of movement. There is a lot of diagonal movement in her nose and eyebrows, yet her eyes and mouth are rounder in shape, making the combination of her features more soft and angled. For her, a print that has some softer lines that move in more of an angled manner, like the print she is wearing, is a smart choice.

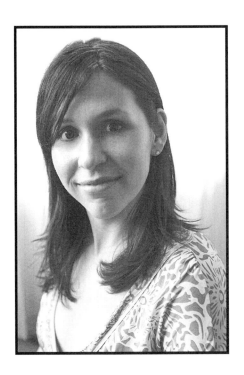
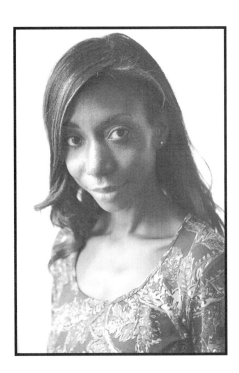

Evaluating your own facial movement

Figuring out how your features move is a bit more complicated than figuring out their texture and intensity level. Some people have obvious features that are very angular, geometric, or soft and round. If this is the case with you, diagnosing your own facial movement will be a bit easier. For most people it isn't that straightforward, so here's a chart to help you. Because it may be overwhelming to look at your face as a whole, it is important to go feature by feature.

EYEBROWS:	Soft and round	Angled	Linear
EYE SHAPE:	Soft and round	Angled	Linear
NOSE SHAPE:	Soft and round	Angled	Linear
MOUTH SHAPE:	Soft and round	Angled	Linear
CHEEK SHAPE:	Soft and round	Angled	Linear

Mark an X on the scale that indicates the movement of each feature. I also recommend that you study a photograph of yourself versus looking in a mirror. It can be challenging to evaluate the movement of your features in person, and by looking at a photo, you can take more time to analyze. You might also want to place a piece of slightly transparent paper, like tracing paper, over the photograph and trace your features to get a better idea of their movement.

For further clarification, here is an example of the chart filled in:

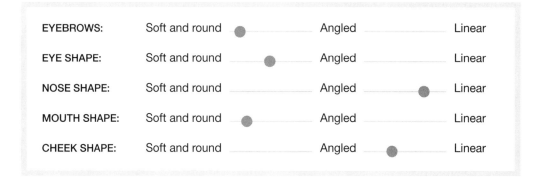

EYEBROWS:	Soft and round	Angled	Linear
EYE SHAPE:	Soft and round	Angled	Linear
NOSE SHAPE:	Soft and round	Angled	Linear
MOUTH SHAPE:	Soft and round	Angled	Linear
CHEEK SHAPE:	Soft and round	Angled	Linear

This person has features that are a combination of soft and more linear. She would look better in prints that move in a more rounded manner but that are also partnered with some linear qualities as well.

If you find that all your features have one type of movement, whether soft and round, angled, or linear, then the best prints for you are ones that have the same movement quality. This does not mean that your entire wardrobe has to be full of round prints or strictly hard geometric patterns. At least make sure that the predominant movement of the print has that quality to it. As a result, you will find that the overall look between you and what you are wearing is much more synergized, helping *you* stand out instead of your prints.

The more variety you have, the more variety you can get away with wearing in your prints. It is important to take note of where the majority of your features fall on the scale and then try to make sure that the majority of movement that your print has moves in that fashion.

Final thoughts on movement

What is most important when it comes to choosing prints?

Choosing prints is very personal and has much to do with our own tastes and style. When considering facial movement as a factor in the decision-making process, it is best to use it as a complement to your personal preferences.

When it comes to print size or scale, there are two things to take into consideration. The first is the size of your features. If you have very large features, then larger prints can work for you. But print size should also be in proportion to your body. You can be a petite person with larger features or a plus-size woman with very small features. So while it is important to always look at your feature size when choosing a print, keep in mind your own body frame as well. The second consideration is personality. I have had very small clients whose personality packs a punch and who can carry off wearing a print that is much larger in scale than their body frames would normally allow for. Other clients who are much larger, and who could presumably wear a larger-scale print, often can't, and they look better in smaller and more demure prints.

Facial movement is one more tool to use when you go shopping. Have I ever broken my own print rule with myself or my clients? Of course I have. Regard this as a guide instead of the gospel.

Finally, trust your gut. When I share information like this with clients, it often confirms gut feelings they had all along. I hear comments like, "Oh, now I understand why that geometric print looked horrible on me." What I always tell my clients and what I'm telling you now is, trust your gut because it's usually right.

Necklines

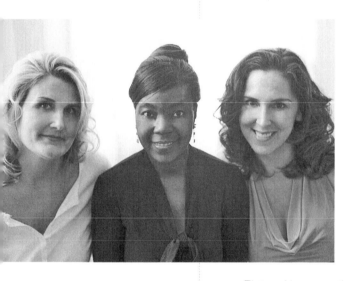

WHETHER I AM speaking in front of a group of women or working privately with a client, I often get asked to help choose a flattering neckline. Many women notice how different certain necklines look on their body, but few women understand why. This section is going to talk about understanding how to choose the most flattering neckline shapes for you.

Pictured here are three women who obviously have very different jawline shapes. The model on the left has a very wide, square-shaped jawline. The model in the middle has a jawline that is as wide as that of the model on the left, but it is much rounder and softer. The model on the right has a much narrower jawline because it is much sharper and tapered-looking.

Being able to recognize your jawline shape is the determining factor in choosing the most flattering neckline.

The rules of choosing neckline shapes

When you repeat the shape of your jawline in your neckline, your jawline gets enhanced or emphasized. This is not necessarily a bad thing; however, many women who do this find that they look unbalanced or that this type of neckline doesn't look good on them. If you want to create a more balanced appearance in your face, choosing a neckline that is the opposite of the shape of your face will do that.

Let's look at some examples.

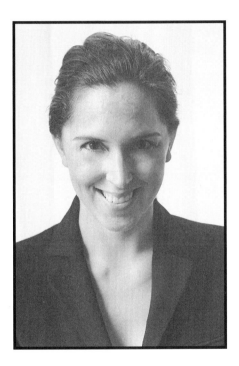 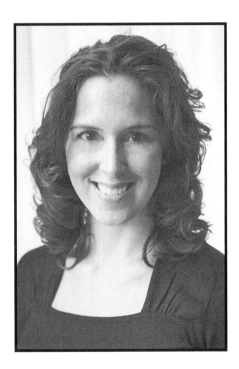

The model pictured above has a very tapered and narrow jawline. In the photo on the left, she is wearing a jacket that mirrors the shape of her jawline, with an opening that is just as narrow and angular as the shape of her chin. In fact, the shape of her chin and the shape of her jawline are practically a perfect match. Because her chin is mirrored in her neckline, the narrowness of her chin is emphasized.

In the photo on the right, her neckline is much more open and wide. Because more space has been opened up around her chin by putting her in a wider neckline, her jawline looks wider and her face looks more balanced.

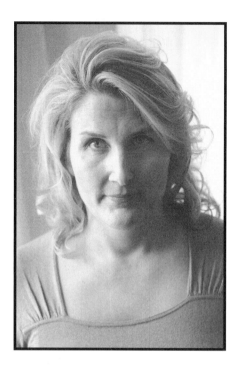 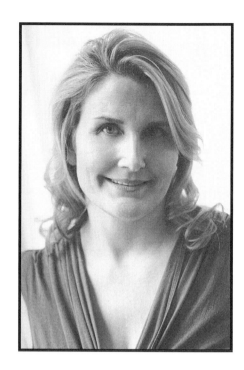

The model pictured here has a very angular and wide jawline. Having such a square jawline, our model's face looks even blunter with a neckline that is also square and mirrors the reflection of her jawline, like the one pictured on the left. Unlike our last model, who had a more tapered jawline and looked more balanced in a wider and squarer neckline, this model's jawline looks wider and more angular.

Wearing a deeper V-neckline, like the one in the photo on the right, does a few things to help balance the jawline. First, the deeper V-neck elongates the overall look of her face, which makes it look longer instead of wider and squarer. Second, the V-neck tapers the shape of her wider and more angular jawline, creating a more balanced overall appearance.

The model pictured here has a jawline with a rounder and wider curved shape to it. In the photo on the left, the rounder neckline mirrors the shape of her jawline, making her face look rounder, wider, and fuller.

By simply putting our model in a top that sits closer to her neck and has a deeper V-shaped neckline, the wideness of her jawline is tapered and narrowed. As a result, her face looks more balanced and less wide and short.

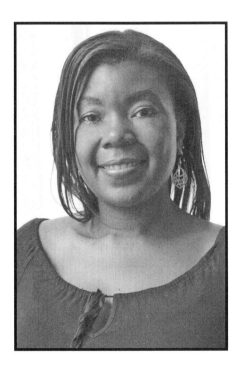
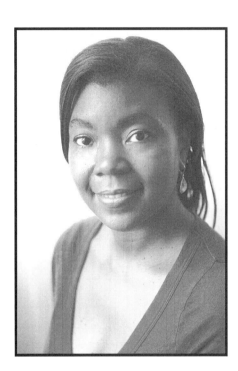

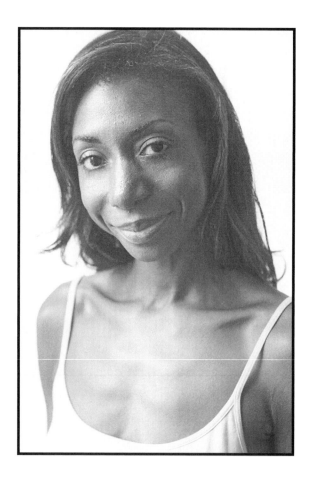

Not only is neckline shape important, but the depth of a neckline matters as well. You may have found that some necklines just look funny, not because of their shape but because of an unflattering depth. When the depth of a neckline doesn't look right, you don't have to throw the shirt away; instead, you can use accessories to make your neckline look more balanced.

In this photo, our model is wearing a flattering neckline shape for her tapered jawline, but the neckline looks too deep and sits too low on her body.

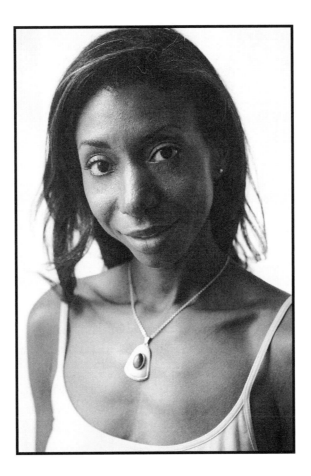

Here the model is wearing the same top, but by simply adding a necklace in that open space between her jaw and her neckline, her face and neckline look more balanced, and there is more synergy between her face and what she is wearing. A necklace can always help balance a neckline that isn't flattering on you.

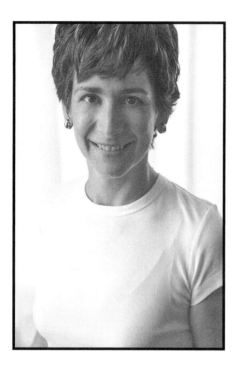
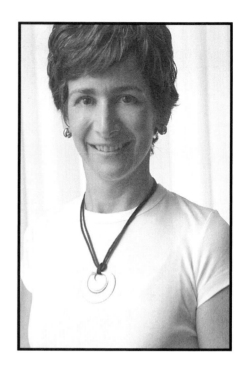

Let's take another look at how a necklace can fix the problem of an unflattering neckline.

On the left, you see our model in a basic crewneck T-shirt. The neckline is a bit high for her neck, causing it to look awkward. On the right, you can see how a simple long necklace draws the eye downward so you don't focus as heavily on how unflattering the neckline is. Because the neckline was not balanced to her face, the use of the necklace creates a more balanced overall appearance.

Find your own flattering neckline shape

Use the following chart to record the shape of your jawline.

JAWLINE:	Tapered	Round	Square

Here is an example of the chart filled out:

JAWLINE:	Tapered	Round	●	Square

Because this person has a jawline that is between a rounder and a squarer shape, she should choose deeper necklines that sit closer to her neck. A wider jaw, either round or square, is elongated and narrowed by a neckline of this style. If she wants to enhance her wider jawline, then she should choose a style that has a rounder or softer square shape.

Tapered, round, and square are the three extremes that your jawline can be. Most people have an oval shaped jawline, which would fall somewhere between tapered and round.

Final thoughts on necklines

What about turtlenecks?

When I discuss necklines with clients, I often get asked about turtlenecks and collared shirts. It is important to point out here that we are talking about necklines, not collared shirts. A turtleneck is a collared shirt, and whether or not a turtleneck or collared shirt is flattering on you has more to do with your neck length than it does with jawline shape. If you want to know more about collared shirts or turtlenecks, review the sections on short and long necks, which will give you all the information you need on choosing these styles.

Are there wrong necklines for me?

Choosing a flattering neckline shape has more to do with personal choice than it does with set rules. Some people want to emphasize the shape of their jawline while others may want to use necklines to bring the shape of the jawline into balance. By using the information in this section, you will be able to make your own choice.

Instead of saying there is a right and a wrong neckline for you based on your jawline shape, you can decide for yourself what you want to enhance or minimize.

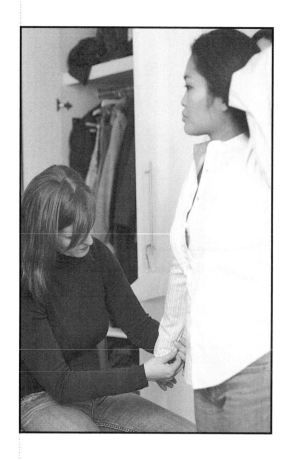

PART III

The CASE
Studies

WHEN CHOOSING THE right clothing, not only will you need to look at your particular body challenges and assets as well as your facial features, but you'll also need to look at your body as a whole to achieve total balance. While diagnosing your body characteristics is a very effective first step, this part will guide you through that final and important last step: bringing it all together.

For each model, I'll diagnose challenges and identify assets. I don't want you to look at the jeans and T-shirt shots as the "before" photos, implying that each model looks bad or wrong in these outfits. Choosing a uniform jeans and T-shirt look simply put the models on a level playing field.

Following each jeans and T-shirt shot will be an outfit that brings it all together. As you look at these case studies, consider what strategies you may be able to use the next time you get dressed.

As you've probably noticed by now, every one of the models in this book has totally different and unique body characteristics that make up her overall shape. You may also find your body to be a close match to one of our models, or you may share several combined body characteristics from one model and a few from another. Either way, you will find this part a great final step to ensure that you are making the right clothing choices, that you'll be able to dress your body as a whole, and that you'll have a great overall and finished look.

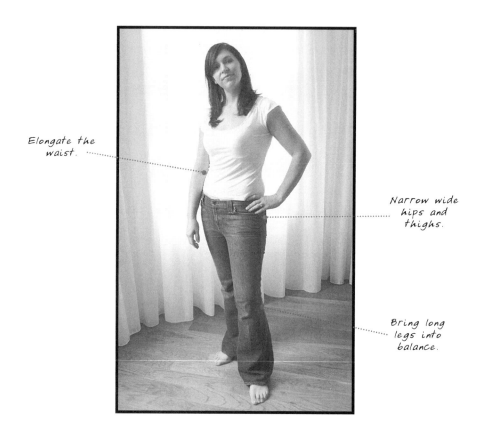

Elongate the waist.

Narrow wide hips and thighs.

Bring long legs into balance.

At five-eleven, our model is very tall, and the majority of her height is in the length of her legs. Her waist is short and overemphasized with such long legs. Her hips are also wide, and she carries the majority of her weight in the bottom half of her body. To bring her body into a more balanced look, the strategy is to lengthen the appearance of her waist, narrow the look of her hips, and shorten the look of her legs.

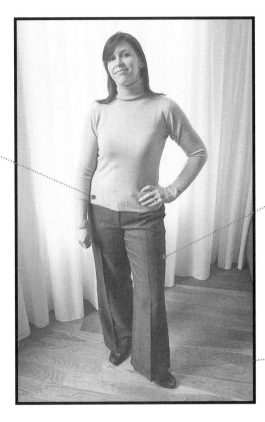

The waist is lengthened with a longer top.

The hips are narrowed and legs are shortened with wider-leg pants.

The legs are shortened with a cuffed pant.

Because our model has so much height, in using pants with a wider leg, we solve two body issues. First, pants that hang straight from the widest part of the hips camouflage the width of the area. Keep in mind that this strategy works only when the top that is being worn has shape in it, like the one she is wearing here. If there weren't any shape in her sweater, she would look boxy and wide. The shape in the sweater gives her a balanced and shaped appearance.

Additionally, because the top she is wearing hits two to three inches below her actual hipbones, the top half of her body is visually lengthened, which makes the top and bottom halves of her body look more balanced with one another.

Women with long legs can also get away with cuffed pants. Horizontal lines placed in an area of the body shorten that area, so the cuffs of these pants break up the length of the leg and make her legs look shorter.

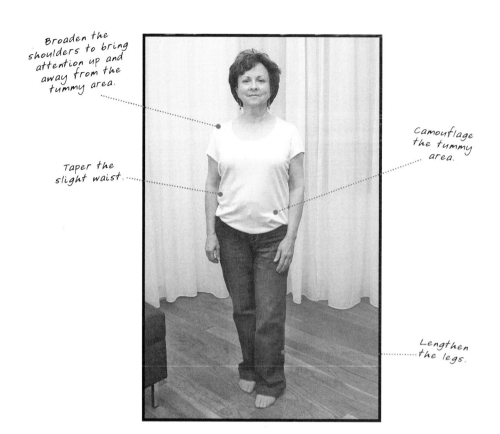

Broaden the shoulders to bring attention up and away from the tummy area.

Taper the slight waist.

Camouflage the tummy area.

Lengthen the legs.

When you are shorter than five-two, like this model, every bit of length counts. The first strategy to balancing her look is to create a longer, leaner line that will elongate and help give her a taller and slimmer appearance. She also collects the majority of her weight in her midsection, so that area of the body is going to be slimmed out through shape and, as a result, bring the attention up toward her face and shoulders and away from her stomach.

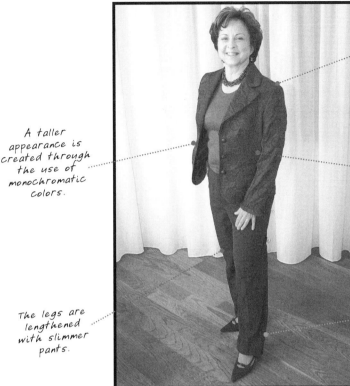

The shoulders are broadened with a jacket that has a strong shoulder line.

A taller appearance is created through the use of monochromatic colors.

The waist is slimmed and defined with a shaped jacket and top.

The legs are lengthened with slimmer pants.

The legs are elongated with pointy-toed shoes that match the color of the pants.

When you are petite, the closer and more fitted your clothing, the taller you will appear. Clothing that is wide shortens and squats the body (and makes it appear wider), so the last thing a petite woman should wear is a big billowy piece of clothing that makes her look shorter. The slimmer pant leg makes our model look taller and slimmer, and the crease elongates the leg because it runs vertically. The pointier toe on the shoe that matches the color of the pants also has an elongating effect.

To avoid bringing the attention to her midsection, instead of camouflaging the area with a shapeless top or jacket, a slimmer and more shaped top and jacket give definition to the area and make her look leaner and taller. The stronger shoulder in the jacket brings the eye up toward her shoulders and face and away from her tummy area.

Lastly, monochromatic dressing elongates her body and makes her look slimmer and taller.

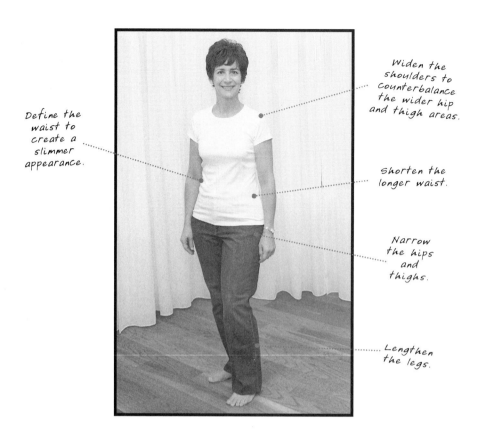

Define the waist to create a slimmer appearance.

Widen the shoulders to counterbalance the wider hip and thigh areas.

Shorten the longer waist.

Narrow the hips and thighs.

Lengthen the legs.

Like most women, our model here collects the majority of her weight throughout her hips, thighs, and butt area. Because she has such narrow shoulders, her body can look very bottom heavy. The goal with her is to increase the width of her shoulders, better define and shorten her waist, taper and elongate her shorter legs, and narrow her wider hip and thigh areas in order to balance her look.

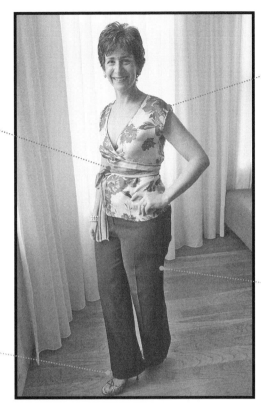

The longer waist is shortened and well defined through the belted top.

The shoulders are widened with a cap sleeve.

Legs are elongated and slimmed with a higher heel.

Wide hips and thighs are minimized with pants that fall straight from her hips.

Most women who collect their weight in their hips and thighs have a much smaller waist. Don't bypass this area: use it. If you don't take advantage of the slimness of your waist, you will wind up looking as wide as your hips. By cinching in our model's waist with a belted top, her look is more proportioned and balanced. Additionally, because horizontal lines shorten an area, the belt does double duty by shortening her long waist, which is naturally long.

Choosing pants that have a straight leg and hang straight from the widest point of her hips

helps to minimize her hips and thighs. Had this pant leg had too much of a peg or tapered hem, it would have emphasized her wider thighs, butt, and hips.

Putting higher heels on our model serves two purposes. First, they elongate the look of the legs (an effect that's also enhanced because the shoe color is close to that of her pants). Second, because of the elongation of the legs with higher heels, the hips and thighs look slimmer.

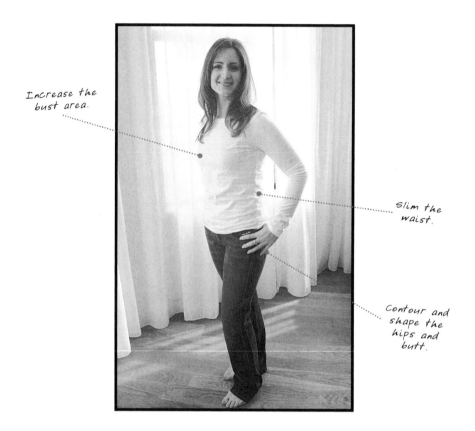

Increase the bust area.

Slim the waist.

Contour and shape the hips and butt.

With a practically straight body from head to toe, this model is ready for some curves. With the model's smaller chest, slight waist, and flatter butt, the strategy is to increase her bustline, taper and define her waist, widen and curve the shape of her hips, and shape and emphasize her butt.

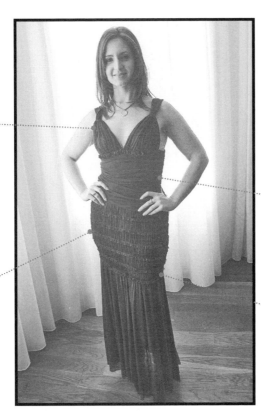

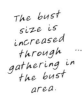

The bust size is increased through gathering in the bust area.

The waist area is defined through shape in the waist.

The hips are widened through horizontal lines.

A curvier appearance is created through the fit-and-flare style of the dress.

Vavavavoom! It took only one dress for our model to go from long and straight to curvy and voluptuous. The dress chosen has a few key features that help achieve this.

First, the gathering at the bust increases the fullness of her chest. Anytime you add gathers to the bust area, it builds up the area by creating a fuller shape. The more defined waist is cinched through shaping in the waist area. Additionally, by increasing the shape of her hip area through the horizontal lines of the skirt, her waist also appears smaller. The fit-and-flare shape in the skirt portion of the dress gives her more of a rounded hip shape and ultimately makes her look a lot curvier.

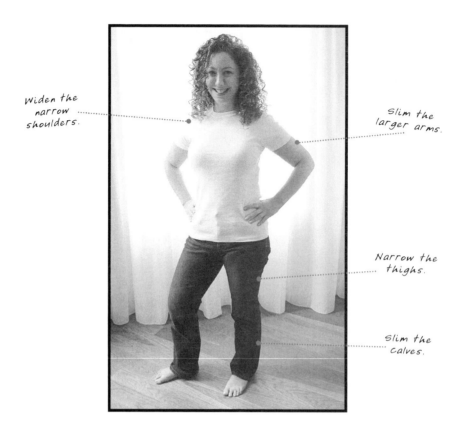

Widen the narrow shoulders.

Slim the larger arms.

Narrow the thighs.

Slim the calves.

Even though our model is a petite size 6, her body has a lot of curve and fullness. Her arms are larger; she collects a good amount of her weight in her thighs and hips, which makes her appear curvier; and she also has larger calves. The strategy here is to contain and mold the curviness of her body with clothing that shapes and balances the curves she does have. Additionally, because her shoulders are very narrow and her hips and thighs much wider, she will look more balanced when her shoulders are widened. This strategy will move the focus off her thigh area and more toward her face.

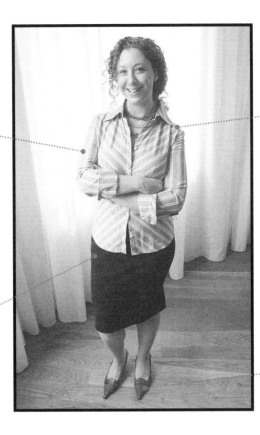

The arms are slimmed with vertical stripes.

The shoulders are widened with diagonal lines that angle outward.

The larger thighs are contained in a skirt that tapers and has structured shape.

The calves are slimmed with pointy-toed shoes.

The goal with our model is to shape the curve that she does have so that she looks curvy as opposed to shapeless. The best way to do this is to choose clothing that sits close to the body and moves with the natural curviness of her body, which will create a slimmer and more balanced look as well. To do this, we used a structured skirt that contains our model's larger thighs. Also, the fact that the skirt tapers or pegs at the hem helps to create a longer and slimmer appearance.

Widening the shoulder area with diagonal stripes that move in an outward direction has two effects. First, the shoulders look broader, which brings focus away from her thigh area. Second, a wider shoulder counterbalances the width of the thighs.

Her larger arms are slimmed with vertical lines, and because our model has larger, curvier calves, a pointier shoe that is lighter in color elongates the look of the leg and makes her calves appear leaner.

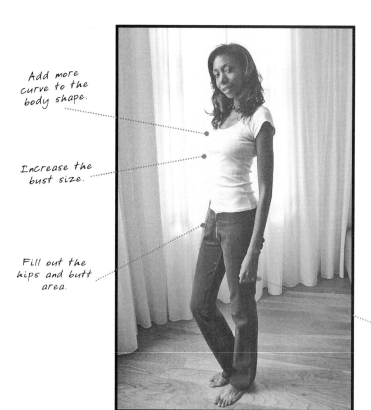

Add more curve to the body shape.

Increase the bust size.

Fill out the hips and butt area.

Shorten the body proportions.

There is certainly nothing wrong with being long and lean, but many long and lean women wish they had a bit more curve. In our model's case, the goal was to create a curvier appearance—one that was a bit more filled out—and to give more shape and fullness to her long lean body.

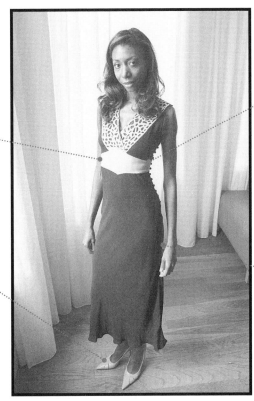

The bust looks fuller with an empire waist.

A long, lean body is shortened and looks fuller with horizontal lines.

Legs are shortened with contrasting-colored shoes.

A curvier shape is created with a fit-and-flare skirt.

Monochromatic dressing makes people look taller, but something as simple as a white band placed horizontally across the waist of this dress makes our model look shorter and therefore fuller in appearance. Additionally, horizontals create width, so the band also makes our model look wider and more shaped. Because the placement of this horizontal line is right below her bustline, fullness is created, making her bust look bigger and curvier.

Choosing a shoe color that contrasts with her skin makes her legs look shorter and breaks up the length of her body, ultimately making her look curvier and more filled out. The fit-and-flare skirt hugs the hips and then flares out at the hem to create more of a rounded and curvier hip shape, which makes her look more voluptuous.

It is common for very slim women to choose big bulky clothing to try to look bigger. However, when bulkier clothing is worn, slim women just look like they are too small for their clothing. Instead, shaped clothing that sits close to the body can create the curved and fuller look many slim women desire.

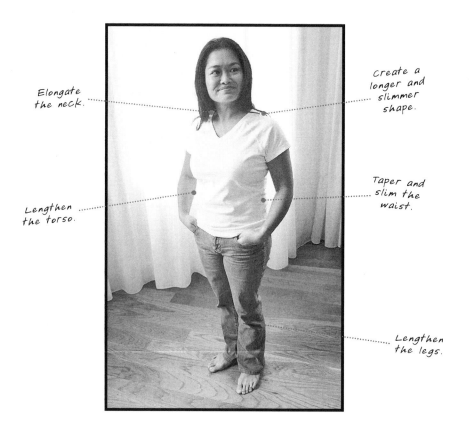

Elongate
the neck.

create a
longer and
slimmer
shape.

Lengthen
the torso.

Taper and
slim the
waist.

Lengthen
the legs.

Our model is very petite, and she looks even shorter because many of her body characteristics are also very short. She has a short neck, waist, and legs. Also, because she doesn't have much of a defined waistline, the goal is to shape her waist, which will also help her appear taller and leaner.

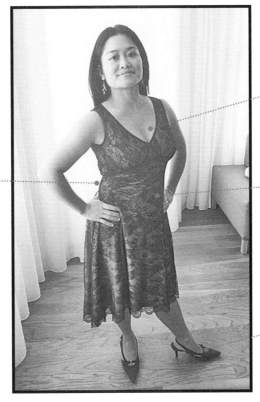

The neck is elongated with a deeper V-neck.

A longer, slimmer overall shape is created through shape in the dress.

The torso appears longer because the dress has no defined waistline.

The legs look longer with pointy-toed shoes.

Oftentimes a petite woman feels like she looks short in a very long dress or skirt. One of the solutions is to have an asymmetrical or uneven hem. This dress is longer in the back so she appears taller.

In addition, the shaping in the dress gives her the illusion of a more shaped and tapered waist, which is also enhanced by the flare shape of the skirt of the dress. The deeper V-neck of the dress opens up her neck area and makes her neck appear longer. Since the dress is one color, there is no intrusion of another color to break up the length of the dress; therefore, her body looks longer. Her shorter torso is also elongated because the waist is bypassed with no clear waist definition in the dress. The pointy-toed shoes also make her legs appear longer.

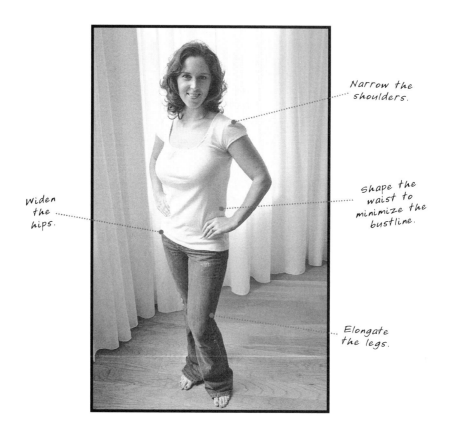

Narrow the
shoulders.

Shape the
waist to
minimize the
bustline.

Widen
the
hips.

Elongate
the legs.

Even at five-seven, it is possible to have short legs, and the model pictured here is a perfect example. In addition, she carries much of her weight on top, with a larger chest and broader shoulders in contrast to her narrow hips. The strategy is to narrow the shoulders and minimize the bustline, and lengthen the look of her legs and widen and create fullness in the bottom half of her body, which will automatically counterbalance and taper the fullness she has on top.

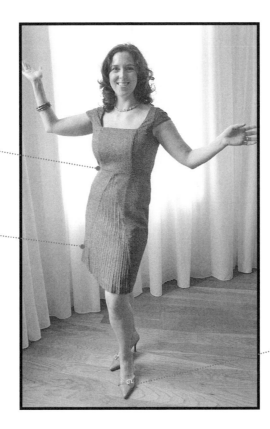

The bust is minimized through shaping in the waist.

A fuller skirt widens the hips and narrows the shoulders.

The legs are elongated with shoes that match the skin color.

By creating fullness though a fuller skirt, the shoulder area and bustline are slimmed. In this model's case, however, the skirt should not be too full because her legs are short. The chosen dress has just enough flair to taper the shoulders and widen the hips without shortening the legs. In addition, her legs appear longer because the color of her shoes matches her skin tone.

The shape of the dress is also important to point out. Because there is shape in the waist, her bustline automatically gets minimized. Had this dress been shapeless or lacking a defined waist, she would have looked top-heavy. The fit-and-flare style creates a much more balanced and proportioned look.

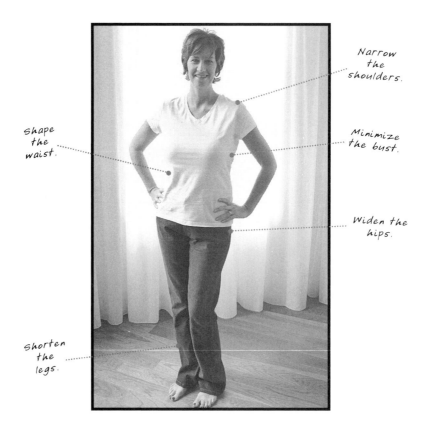

Narrow
the
shoulders.

Minimize
the bust.

Shape
the
waist.

Widen the
hips.

Shorten
the
legs.

The tall model pictured here has long legs. She also has very broad shoulders, a large chest, and narrow hips, which make her body appear very big and wide on top. There are several strategies that can be implemented to make her body appear more balanced and proportioned: Minimize the width of her shoulders, shape the waist, minimize the bust, widen her hips, and shorten the look of her legs.

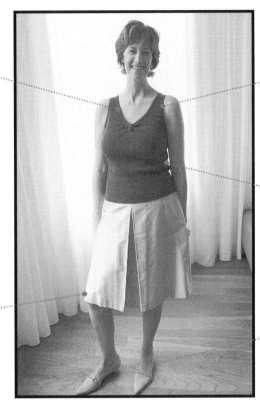

The bust is minimized with a deeper V.

The shoulders are narrowed with an armhole that cuts inward.

The bustline is minimized with shaping in the waist.

The legs are shortened, the shoulders are narrowed, and the waist is more defined with a fuller skirt.

The legs are shortened with flatter shoes.

The taller you are and the longer your legs, the fuller the skirt you can wear. As you can see, the fullness of this skirt shortens the length of her legs. The skirt paired with a flatter shoe makes our model's legs look shorter.

Additionally, the crisp fullness of the skirt increases the width of her hips, which slims the width of her shoulders, gives her more of a defined waist, and minimizes her bust size. The angled neckline also tapers her shoulders. You

may notice gathering in the neckline, but because that gathering is not located directly on her bustline, it has a minimal effect on the size of her chest.

Because our model has such a large chest, shaping the waist is important. If this top lacked defined shape in the waist, her body would look much boxier when worn with such a full skirt. The shape of the top is creating more of a balance between the top and bottom halves of her body.

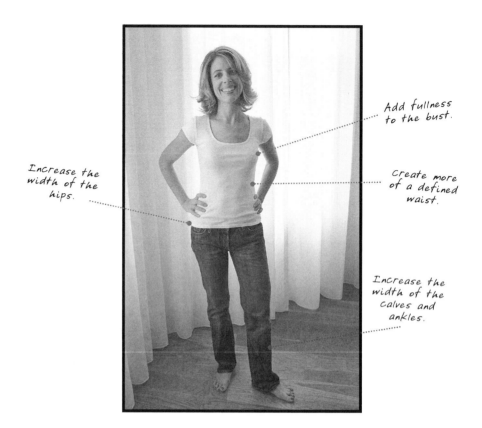

Add fullness
to the bust.

Increase the
width of the
hips.

Create more
of a defined
waist.

Increase the
width of the
calves and
ankles.

The model pictured here is narrow and slim. She has a smaller chest; little waist definition; and narrow, straighter hips. The strategy is to use clothing to create a body that has more curve and shape through fullness in the right places and shape in others.

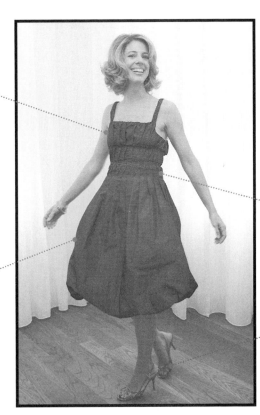

A fuller bust is created with shaped gathering in the bust area.

The waist is defined with shape in the waist and a fuller skirt.

The hip area is widened with a fuller skirt.

The calves and ankles look fuller with a darker shoe.

Our model is wearing a dress that creates fullness in the right places without her getting lost in the effect.

The detailed, shaped gathering in her bust area creates the look of a fuller chest. Her waist is cinched, and this shape defines it. The crisp gathers in the skirt give this piece tremendous volume, which helps give her a fuller hip area. This fullness in the skirt also makes her waist appear more tapered.

The fact that her shoe color doesn't match her skin tone makes her legs appear heavier. It may seem that the last thing a woman would want to do is make her calves and ankles appear larger, but it is an important shoe choice because the fullness of the skirt, which enhances her hip size, also makes her legs appear slimmer. Our model has such thin ankles and calves that she benefits by using a darker shoe to help them appear fuller.

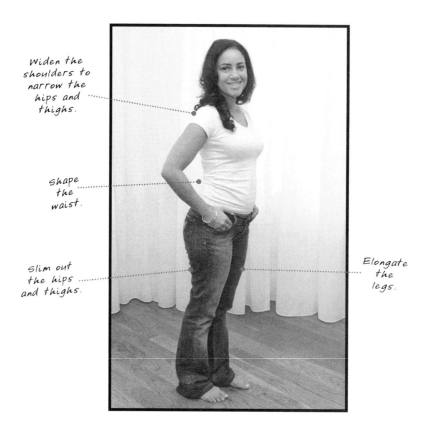

Widen the shoulders to narrow the hips and thighs.

Shape the waist.

Slim out the hips and thighs.

Elongate the legs.

The model pictured here is all curves. She has fuller thighs and hips and a rounder butt. The strategy for her is to balance this shape in clothing that sits close to the body and that works with her curves instead of fighting them. She has a defined waist that shouldn't be bypassed with shapeless clothing, which will only make her look shapeless. In addition, she is very petite with short legs, so adding length to her body will also taper her curves and elongate her body without covering up the natural curves she was born with.

Hips and thighs are counterbalanced and slimmed with a wider neckline.

The waist is slimmed with shaping that creates an overall slimmer appearance.

Legs are elongated with a pointier shoe that matches the color of her pants.

Larger hips, thighs, and butt are counterbalanced and minimized by boot-cut pants.

One of the subtlest points of this outfit is how much shape there is in the sweater. Had there been no shape in the top, she would have no defined waist, and her whole body would look like a straight line that is as wide as her bust and hips. With a cinch of the waist through a more shaped sweater, she looks perfectly balanced and curved.

The wider neckline and boot-cut pants counterbalance the natural curve of her body and therefore bring the focus away from her wider thighs and hips without camouflaging or covering them up.

The pointier shoe that she has on makes her legs appear longer, and the fact that they match the color of her pants creates a longer and slimmer leg that also tapers the width of her thighs.

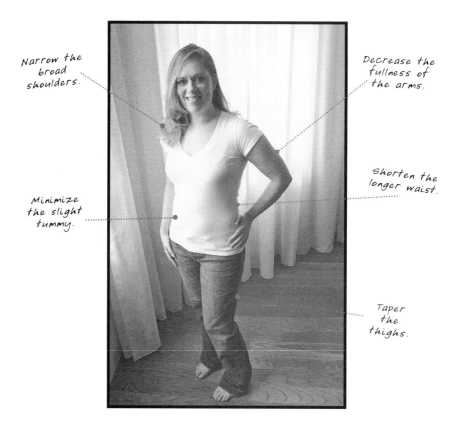

Narrow the broad shoulders.

Decrease the fullness of the arms.

Minimize the slight tummy.

Shorten the longer waist.

Taper the thighs.

The model pictured here has fuller arms and broad shoulders; a longer waist; and fuller thighs, hips, and butt. She also has a slight tummy. The strategy with her is to taper and narrow her shoulders and arms, shorten her waist, and minimize the fullness that's in her tummy, hips, thighs, and butt.

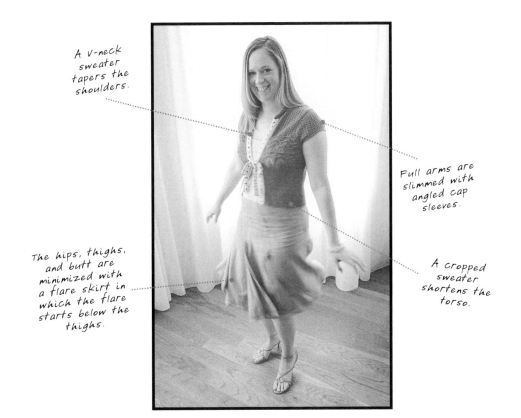

A v-neck sweater tapers the shoulders.

Full arms are slimmed with angled cap sleeves.

The hips, thighs, and butt are minimized with a flare skirt in which the flare starts below the thighs.

A cropped sweater shortens the torso.

After everything I have said, it may seem strange to put a full skirt on someone who has large thighs, but there are a few things going on with this skirt that work. The fullness of the skirt starts below her thighs, which make her hips, thighs, and butt look smaller. If the fullness of the skirt had started right below the waist, that area would have looked bigger.

The shaped, cropped sweater shortens the longer waist. It is important that the sweater the model is wearing is shaped and sits close to her body. Without that definition, she would look boxier and wide.

The deeper V closure of the sweater angles and narrows her wider shoulders, and the angling of the cap sleeve has a slimming effect on her arms.

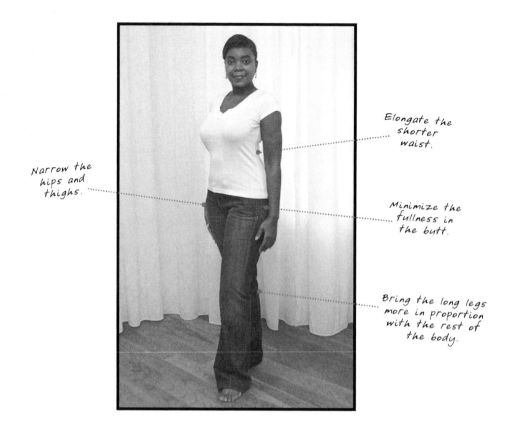

Elongate the shorter waist.

Narrow the hips and thighs.

Minimize the fullness in the butt.

Bring the long legs more in proportion with the rest of the body.

The model pictured here is very curvy. The strategy here is to choose clothing that moves with the shape of her natural curve. She is also very short-waisted, with legs that are much longer in proportion to the rest of her body. As a result, she looks squat on top.

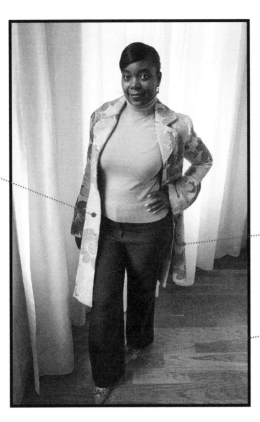

The torso looks longer and the legs look shorter with a longer jacket.

The butt, hips, and thighs are minimized with a longer, shaped jacket.

The legs are shortened with a shoe that doesn't match the color of the pants.

A long jacket is the saving grace for many women who collect their weight in their hips, thighs, and butt. There are a few rules to follow when choosing a long jacket successfully, and this one is a good example. First, there is shape in the jacket. A long jacket without shape will just make you look boxy. Second, the length is long enough that her hips and thighs are completely covered up. Lastly, at five-seven, our model is tall enough to pull off wearing a jacket with so much length. I wouldn't suggest a longer jacket if you are petite or have short legs.

From Part I of this book, you may remember that this model has a short neck, making a turtleneck seem like a bad choice for her. While a turtleneck isn't always the best choice, the long line created by the jacket creates an elongating effect and helps achieve balance. In addition, she is wearing shorter earrings, which have an elongating effect on shorter necks.

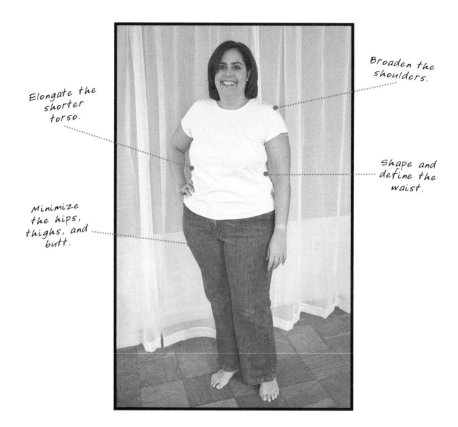

Broaden the
shoulders.

Elongate the
shorter
torso.

Shape and
define the
waist.

Minimize
the hips,
thighs, and
butt.

Our model here has very narrow shoulders, which enhance the fact that she collects the majority of her weight in her hips, butt, and thighs. The goal is to widen her shoulders, which will counterbalance the fullness in the lower half of her body; minimize her hips, butt, and thigh area; and define her slimmer waist, which will give her an overall slimmer appearance. Her arms are also very long (her thumb knuckle hangs lower than her crotch), and her torso is very short. So the focus is also on elongating her torso and shortening the look of her arms.

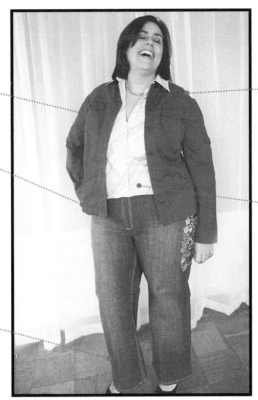

The shoulders are widened with eye-catching patch pockets.

The torso is elongated with a jacket that is longer than the shirt.

The hips, thighs, and butt are minimized with a straighter jean that doesn't peg or taper at the hem.

The shoulders are broadened with a strong shoulder line on the jacket.

The waist is defined and slimmed with diagonal stripes in the shirt and defined shaping in the waist of the jacket.

In this photo, the shoulder is built up though the stronger shoulder line in the jacket. The patch pockets bring the attention up toward the shoulder, and the horizontal line of the top opening of the patch pockets visually widens her shoulder line. This stronger line offers many advantages to her overall look. Because her shoulder is widened, it counterbalances the fullness in her hips, butt, and thighs, making them look more tapered and balanced with the rest of her body. In addition, her hips, butt, and thighs are also minimized because her jeans aren't narrow or tapered at the hem. Her jeans fall straighter from the widest point of her hips, which slims her legs. Wearing a heel also has an elongating and, therefore, slimming effect on her larger thighs.

The diagonal stripes in her shirt have a slimming effect on her waist, and the shaped jacket defines her waist, giving her a more balanced and slimmer appearance overall.

The jacket is longer than the shirt, drawing the eye downward and lengthening her shorter torso.

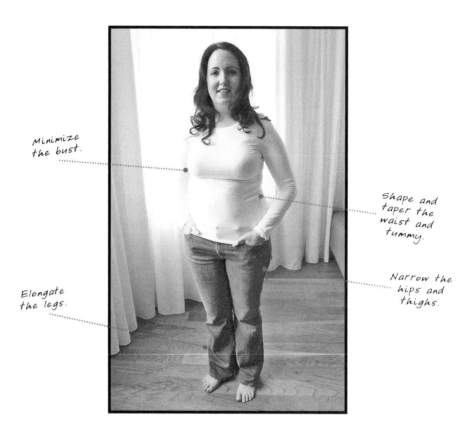

Minimize
the bust.

Shape and
taper the
waist and
tummy.

Narrow the
hips and
thighs.

Elongate
the legs.

The model in this photo is wider in her waist as well as her hips and thighs. The main strategy with her was to slim out her tummy and thighs, which would also create a longer and slimmer body. This model is also petite at five-two and has shorter legs, so creating a longer line will not only slim her tummy, thighs, and hips but also help her appear taller. The focus is to also balance the fullness of her bustline.

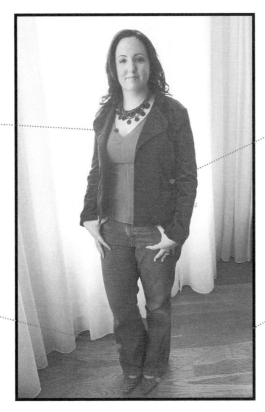

The bust is minimized with a deep V-neck.

The body is elongated with a shaped jacket and top.

The thigh and hip area are counterbalanced with a boot-cut pant.

The legs appear longer with a slight heel and narrower shoe with a pointier toe.

By taking the emphasis away from her midsection through the shaping of a jacket and top, you can see how the model's hips and thighs are automatically slimmed and tapered. This is because the focus is no longer on the width of her midsection. By shaping her waist, an overall longer and leaner look is achieved. The deeper V-neckline has a minimizing effect on her larger chest.

Instead of choosing a shoe that is completely flat, the shoe she is wearing has a slight heel. Even if it is the smallest of heels, it will always help make the legs look longer and therefore leaner.

When a body has areas that are wide and you are petite, the best thing to do is to slim those areas through shaping and wearing clothing that sits closer to the body. You score doubly by not only slimming the area but making the body appear to be longer than it actually is.

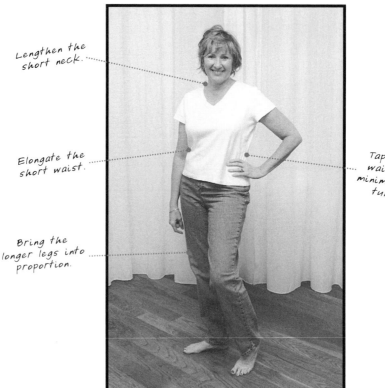

Lengthen the short neck.

Elongate the short waist.

Taper the waist and minimize the tummy.

Bring the longer legs into proportion.

In this photo, you can see what happens when a shorter, less-shaped cropped top is worn by someone who has a shorter waist. Her waist looks short. The strategy here is to elongate her torso and slim out her wider waist and slight tummy.

It may also surprise some people that petite women can have extremely long legs. Believe it or not, long legs are not just found on tall women. Our model at five-three has very long legs, but being petite, we want to give her every bit of length we can. So the goal isn't necessarily to shorten her legs but to elongate her torso so that it appears to be in proportion with her legs.

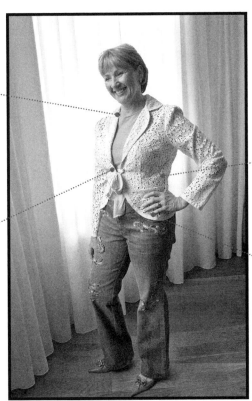

The neck is elongated with a lighter-colored top that closely matches the skin color.

The waist is shaped with a shaped jacket.

The torso is elongated with a jacket that has a deeper, lower closure.

The tummy is minimized with a fit-and-flare jacket.

Because this jacket closes lower on the body, the torso appears to be longer. Additionally, the fit-and-flare style of the jacket shapes her waist and camouflages her tummy.

The color of the top almost matches her skin tone. Because of this, her neck looks longer and her waist also looks elongated. If you have a short neck and want to wear higher necklines, the lighter-colored the top the better.

Her leg length wasn't made shorter because she is petite. Instead of shortening her legs to match her shorter torso, the goal here was to lengthen her torso so that it matched the length of her legs, which not only makes her torso look longer but gives her an overall taller and leaner appearance.

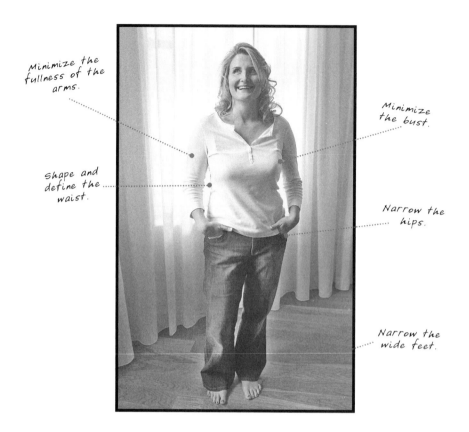

Minimize the fullness of the arms.

Minimize the bust.

Shape and define the waist.

Narrow the hips.

Narrow the wide feet.

In this photo, our model has a much squarer shape from bust to hip. The goal is to taper her waist, minimize her bust, and give her more shape and curve that doesn't enhance the size of her chest. In addition, we want to slim and narrow her hips, arms, and feet, which are naturally fuller on her.

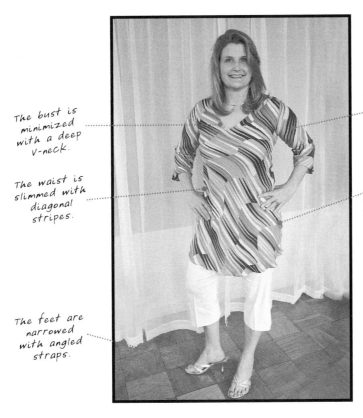

The arms are slimmed with diagonal lines.

The bust is minimized with a deep V-neck.

The waist is slimmed with diagonal stripes.

The bust and waist are minimized with a longer, shaped tunic-style top.

The feet are narrowed with angled straps.

The deeper V-neck of this tunic opens up her bust area, which minimizes the fullness of her chest. In addition, her bust is also minimized because of the longer tunic style she is wearing. A way to make a bustline look smaller is to wear a shaped top that ends two to three inches below the hipbones or lower, which makes anyone with a large chest look less squat and busty. Because our model has height, she can wear such a long top. It is important to point out the

shape in this tunic style as well: had it not shaped our model's waist, it would look boxy and square, which would make her look boxy and square. The diagonal stripes in the print of the tunic shape her waist and therefore give it more definition.

The diagonal stripes on the sleeves taper and slim her fuller arms, and the diagonal stripes on her shoes narrow her very wide feet.

Goodbye Note

IT IS MY hope that this book helped you take a big first step toward what I refer to as becoming "fluent in your own style." While there are many components and facets to creating your own personal style, setting the foundational rules of choosing the right clothing for your body is an important first step upon which everything else is built.

I hope this book has given you a renewed sense of how to choose the right clothing for your body, a feeling of control in an area where you lacked a sense of mastery, and an overall game plan that will make buying and wearing clothing something that you actually consider fun and enjoyable.

Of course, the journey of our own personal style transformation is a winding course and one that is never really over, so I invite all of you to be in touch either personally or through my e-mail newsletter. Feel free to contact me at bridgette@bridgetteraes.com or visit www.bridgetteraes.com for more information.

It has been a pleasure and an honor to be able to share this information with you and to help you all learn how to take the next step in setting your style free.

Glossary

A-LINE SKIRT: A skirt that is wider at the hem and therefore shaped like an A.

ANGLE: Lines in clothing that move in a diagonal or slanted manner and have a slimming effect wherever they are placed on the body.

ANKLE STRAPS: Straps found on a pair of shoes—such as buckles, ties, or strapping—that fasten around the ankle.

BANGLE BRACELET: A solid bracelet that has no movement or flexibility.

BELL SLEEVE: A sleeve that is proportionately wider at the hem, giving it a bell shape.

BILLOWY: A term used to describe clothing made from softer fabrics that has movement and fluidity to it; usually lacking shape and structure.

BOATNECK: A neckline that sits higher on the neck, usually at the clavicle point, and that has a wide opening toward the outer part of the shoulders.

BOUCLÉ: A fabric that is made from uneven yarns that, when woven, are often looped to create a textured and knobby appearance.

BOXY: Used to describe silhouettes that lack shape or structure.

BRACELET-LENGTH SLEEVE: A sleeve that is an inch or two shorter than long sleeves. It's called a bracelet length because it allows room for a bracelet to be seen.

CABLE KNIT SWEATER: A sweater that has a textural knit stitch created by crossing one group of stitches over another, creating the look of a cable.

CAMISOLE: A garment often resembling lingerie, used as a layering piece underneath shirts to protect from sheerness or exposure.

CAP SLEEVE: A short sleeve that covers the shoulder and minimally covers the top part of the arm.

CENTER BACK OUTLET: Excess fabric found inside the back seam of pants and contained within the waistband that allows for letting out and making the pants wider in the waist. This feature is usually found in better-made pants.

CENTER BACK SEAM: The vertical seam that runs down the center of the back of clothing, including skirts, jackets, shirts, and pants.

CENTER BACK WAIST: The middle back of the waist found in all tops, jackets, and dresses, usually with a seam that runs vertically down the center of the garment.

CHANDELIER EARRINGS: Long, decorative earrings that mimic the ornate quality of a chandelier.

CHOKER: A necklace that fastens closely at the base of the neck. Scarves when wound closely to the base of the neck can be tied in a choker fashion.

CINCH: The action of gathering and tightening clothing in a specific area of the body (usually the waist) through shaping in the clothing's natural construction by way of elastic or drawstrings or through the use of a belt or other fastening measures. Example: A shirt is cinched with a belt.

CONTRAST: The difference between colors when placed next to each other. The greater the difference, the greater the contrast. Black and white create a strong contrast, while tan and white have a lower contrast.

COUNTERBALANCE: To oppose an area that is full or wide with fullness at its opposite end.

COWL NECK: A turtleneck style that is more draped and open around the neck.

CREASED LEG: Found in tailored pants; through pressing, a crease is created down the center of a pant leg.

CROPPED PANTS/CAPRI PANTS: Pants that are slightly shorter than full length. The length of capri or cropped pants varies from right below the knee to right above the ankle.

CROPPED SHIRT OR JACKET: A shirt or jacket whose length is shorter than the natural hipbone.

CROTCH POINT: On the body, it is the point where the pelvis ends and the legs begin. On pants, the crotch is where the two legs of the pants join.

DARTS: A tapered and stitched tuck used to create shape in clothing, found in all types of garments.

DIAGONAL LINES: Lines that angle or slant, which have a slimming effect when used in clothing.

DOUBLE-BREASTED: Having a double row of vertically placed buttons that run parallel to one another, usually found on jackets but also on some dresses, skirts, and shirts.

DOUBLE LAYER: Layering two shirts and wearing as one. Usually the lower layer is longer than the outer layer, and the layers are usually two different colors.

DRAPEY FABRICS: Fabrics that are soft and fluid and that, when made into garments, have gentle movement to them.

DROPPED SHOULDER: When the shoulder seam that connects a sleeve to the armhole rests slightly off the shoulder and on the top part of the upper arm instead. Commonly found in more relaxed styles of T-shirts and jackets.

ELONGATE: To make an area appear longer. In clothing, this is often done through shaping and vertical lines.

EPAULETS: A military-inspired shoulder strap of fabric that runs along the shoulder line, used on jackets, dresses, and shirts.

FIT AND FLARE: Found in pants and skirts, a shaped silhouette that tapers at the knee point and then flares out again, making it wider at the hem.

FLAT-FRONT PANTS: Pants that have no pleating or gathering at the front waist area, creating flatness over the tummy area of the pants.

GATHERS/GATHERING: An accumulation of fabric secured by either stitching or elastic, which creates fullness in the garment.

HALTER TOP: A woman's top secured around the neck without any sleeves.

HIPBONE ZONE: Located two to three inches below the hipbone. When a sweater or shirt ends in this zone, the results are often very flattering.

HORIZONTAL LINES: Seam lines that move left to right, found in stripes and cuffs. These lines have a shortening and widening effect when used in clothing.

INTENSITY: The level of sharpness or boldness of coloring, either of a person or in clothing.

LOW-RISE PANTS: Pants that are shorter in length from the crotch to the top of the waist, therefore causing the pants to usually sit lower than one's natural waist.

MARY JANE SHOES: Shoes that have a strap over the instep and usually a more rounded toe, often having a younger, juvenile feel because they are traditionally worn by young girls.

MATTE: Lacking any sheen or shine; a dull surface.

MONOCHROMATIC: Shades or tones of one color.

MOVEMENT: The style by which features or prints move—that is, soft, geometric, or linear.

MUFFIN TOP: An excess bulge that can creep over a waistband of a skirt or pants when the fit of the garment is too tight.

NAPPED FABRIC: A soft raised surface on fabrics such as velvet and corduroy.

NATURAL WAIST: The natural waist point on the body, which varies from person to person and is usually discovered by placing the hands on the waist.

OPTIC: Bold contrasting color combinations.

PEGGED SKIRT: A skirt that tapers or is narrower at the hem.

PENDANT: A style of necklace that has a thin chain or cord with a larger motif hanging from it.

PINSTRIPE: A very thin stripe found in tailored fabrics.

POP COLOR: A bright color that is added to an outfit in a smaller amount for interest and variation, usually found in accent pieces and accessories as well as in shirts and tops.

PRINCESS SEAMS: A curved seam used to give shape to garments, usually found in shirts, dresses, and jackets.

PUFF SLEEVE: A full sleeve that is gathered at the hem.

RAGLAN SLEEVE: An armhole that starts at the neckline and has a slanted shape to it, creating a softer shoulder appearance.

RECOVERY: The amount of bounce back or spring ability found in a stretchy fabric or garment, enabling it to revert back to its original shape. The better spring a stretch fabric or garment has after it has been stretched from wear, the more recovery it has.

RIB: Vertical rows of stitching on a sweater, which often have good natural elasticity.

RUCHING: (pronounced *rooshing*) Another term for gathering.

SHAPE: Clothing that has shaping through elasticity, seaming, or silhouette style.

SHAPELESS TOPS: Tops and sweaters with no defined waist shape.

SHEEN: Luster or shine.

SHIRTTAIL: Found on button-down shirts, a rounded hem traditionally used to more easily tuck in shirts but which can be worn outside the waistband of a skirt or pants.

SHORTEN: The act of making something look visually shorter. In clothing, horizontal lines and wider silhouettes often have a shortening effect.

SIDE SEAM: The seam that runs up and down the side of a garment, and when the clothing is worn, it runs up and down the sides of your body.

SINGLE-BREASTED: A singular row of buttons that runs down the front center of a garment.

SPAGHETTI STRAPS: Thin straps, usually no thicker than one-quarter inch, that go over the shoulder; commonly used on thin tops and dresses.

SPANDEX/LYCRA: A synthetic fiber that is woven into fabric to give it stretch and comfort. Similar to spandex, Lycra is an elastane fiber developed by DuPont.

STRAIGHT-LEG PANTS: Pants that fall straight from the hips and have wider leg openings.

SURFACE INTEREST: Any tactile or three-dimensional qualities in a fabric.

TEXTURE: A tactile quality in a fabric.

TEXTURED WEAVE: A fine woven fabric that has small, sometimes nondescript, surface interest woven into it.

THREE-QUARTER SLEEVE: A sleeve that is no longer than a few inches below the elbow. Frequently found on sweaters, shirts, and jackets.

T-STRAP: A strap on a shoe that runs vertically down the vamp or instep of the foot and connects to an ankle strap, thereby creating the look of a T.

TUNIC: A longer shirt or sweater, either shaped or loose, that hangs at or below the hips.

TWEED: A multicolor irregularly woven fabric that has textural qualities.

VERTICAL LINES: Lines that move up and down, such as pinstripes, ribbed knits, or vertical rows of buttons. Vertical lines have an elongating and slimming effect wherever they are placed on the body.

WRAP TOP: A top or dress that wraps on itself in a real or faux fashion, often with self-belting ties.

Acknowledgments

I MUST TAKE a moment to acknowledge those who made this book happen. Being my first book, it is also a tremendous milestone in my career, so I must also take the opportunity to thank those who helped me get to this point.

To Lori Berkowitz, for being my partner on the journey of creating this book; for your talents, your vision, your commitment, your humor; and for pouring yourself into this book so generously.

To my editor, Meg Leder, for your belief in me, for your excitement and passion for this project, and for cheering me along every step of the way. You are more than an editor; you are my friend.

To my agent, Marilyn Allen, for always going that extra mile and for sticking by me until my voice found a home.

To all the models who participated in this project: Anna Ayers, Benke Davis, Joyce Dollinger, Theresa Exconde-Press, Denise Grant, Jessica Halprin, Tania Kleckner, Makeba Lloyd, Julie Meyer, Jeanmarie

Payne, Cherie Pelowski, Anne Townsend, Nadja Webb, Cara Tuzzalino Werben, Lisa Wilson, Beth Wuhrl, and Marianna Zonenberg. Thank you for lending your beautiful selves, your wonderful spirits, to this book, and for giving it beauty and life. Most important, thank you for your willingness to boldly represent the diversity that we as women share.

To Lauren Andrews, for your work and talents in photography and production, and for being the glue that held everything together during the shooting of the photographs.

To Gaston Olsen, for capturing the real moments of the photo shoot through your candid photography, and for your skilled eye.

To Susan Donoghue and Lauren Whitworth, for lending us your talents in makeup, and to Herman "Jay" Thibodeaux, for your hair artistry.

To Max Studio, for supplying us with much of the clothing used for the photography.

To the most important person in my life and my heart: my husband and best friend, Frank Mazzola. Sharing this with you is my greatest joy. Thank you for your love, for your encouragement, for giving me the room to fulfill my dreams, for your patience and unwavering belief in me. You add the sweetness, fun, and laughter to my life. I love you *ttthhhiiiissss* much.

A special thank-you to my mother, Liz Raes, who taught me that I had every right and ability to create the life that I wanted and then sacrificed, supported, and encouraged me every step of the way. You are a woman of strength and resilience.

To my sister, Beth Wuhrl: You have been my partner through every chapter of my life, and I couldn't imagine you not being a part of this one.

To those who have supported me: Heather Mann, Bryian "Fatty" Davis, Melissa Leonard, Marybeth Ray, Cheryl Cottino, Alicia Mikoloski, Jerry Dellova, Cammi Yamashiro, Anna Ayers, Fabian Lliguin, Lavita McMath-Turner, Deb Townes, Robert DiMauro, Mishel Herrera, Julie Jansen, Karen Rancourt, Lisa Hennig, Kathi Elster, Carolyn Beale, Carole Flaum, Keith Eschenburg, Kate McKee, Marta Kagan, Bill Pellegrino, Croz, Joe Nunziata, Lisa and Larry Wilson, Tamika Hardy, Jennifer Grove, Lisa Zaslow, Stacy Francis, Jennifer Macaluso-Gilmore, Laura Allen, Giella Poblocki, Mercedes Gonzalez, Michelle Madhock, Melissa Tosetti, Mark Montalbano, and Raul Plansencia.

To the incredible women I feel privileged to call my clients. I wouldn't be writing this book if it weren't for all of you. You are my muses and my inspiration. Each of you welcomed me into your closets and your hearts, put your trust in me, and taught me as much as I have taught you. I am nothing but grateful.

Index

About the Author

AFTER TEN YEARS of working as a fashion designer, a life-changing event motivated **Bridgette Raes** to redirect her career to include more empowering work with women. In 2002, Bridgette launched the New York City–based Bridgette Raes Style Group and has since personally transformed the styles of hundreds of women worldwide.

In addition to her private client work, Bridgette's refreshing approach to fashion and style has earned her frequent requests to speak at many women's organizations and major corporations. Her media work has been seen and heard on CNN, *Good Morning America*, and CBS News Radio; her expert insights have been shared in *Women's World Magazine*, the *Boston Globe*, MSN.com, and AOL.com; and her writing has appeared on Modernmom.com, in *Budget Savvy* magazine, and on Shefinds.com, in addition to her own weekly fashion and style newsletter, which has an international subscriber base and a loyal following.

Bridgette received her fashion design degree and image training from the Fashion Institute of Technology and resides in Brooklyn, New York, with her husband, Frank. She can be reached at www.bridgetteraes.com.

About the Photographer

DRAWN INTO PHOTOGRAPHY by a photo-enthusiast father, **Lori Berkowitz** was one of those kids who always had a camera with her. She got her first Canon SLR at age twelve, and she quickly developed an affinity for photographing people.

Lori has spent the last nine years building her reputation as a talented photographer who is capable of handling a variety of jobs for a discerning clientele. In 2001, Gaston Olsen joined her, and the business expanded exponentially. Lori and Gaston capture two different perspectives simultaneously and nothing is missed. Whether it is a high-society wedding, a big-dollar corporate event, a celebrity party, or an A-list social gathering, they are the ones to capture the moments! For more information, please go to www.loriberkowitzphoto.com and have a look.

ORCHID
BASICS

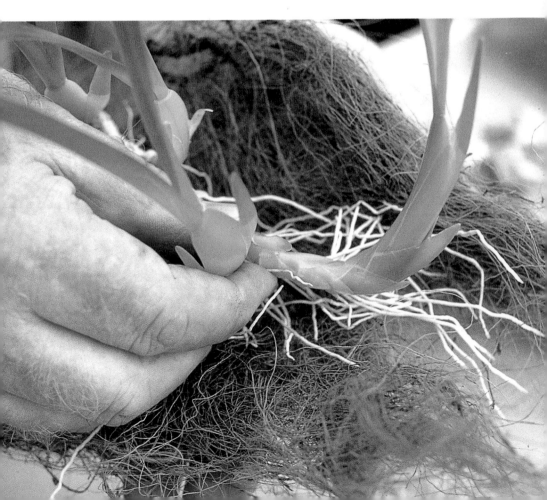

ORCHID

Publishing Director: Alison Goff
Creative Director: Keith Martin
Executive Editor: Julian Brown
Editor: Karen O'Grady
Executive Art Editor: Mark Winwood
Design: Rozelle Bentheim
Picture Research: Sally Claxton
Production Controller: Lucy Woodhead
Cover Photography: Mark Winwood
Illustrator: Martin Jarman

Library of Congress Cataloging-in-Publication Data Available

10 9 8 7 6 5 4 3 2 1

Published by Sterling Publishing Company, Inc.
387 Park Avenue South, New York, NY 10016
First published in Great Britain by Hamlyn, a division of Octopus
Publishing Group Limited
© 2000 Octopus Publishing Group Limited
Distributed in Canada by Sterling Publishing
c/o Canadian Manda Group, One Atlantic Avenue, Suite 105,
Toronto, Ontario, Canada M6K 3E7

Printed in China

Sterling ISBN 0-8069-2289-3

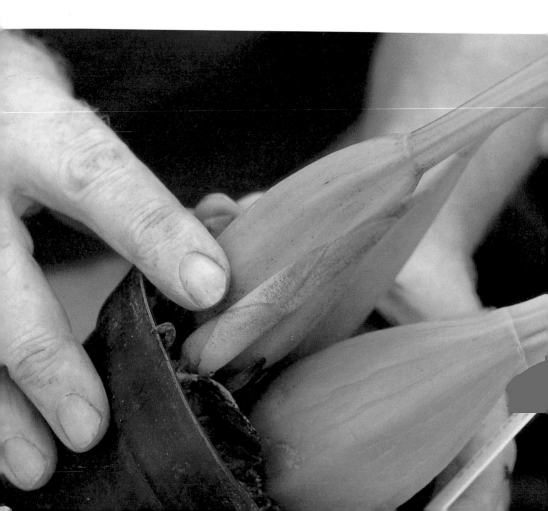

BASICS

Isobyl la Croix

Sterling Publishing Co., Inc.
New York

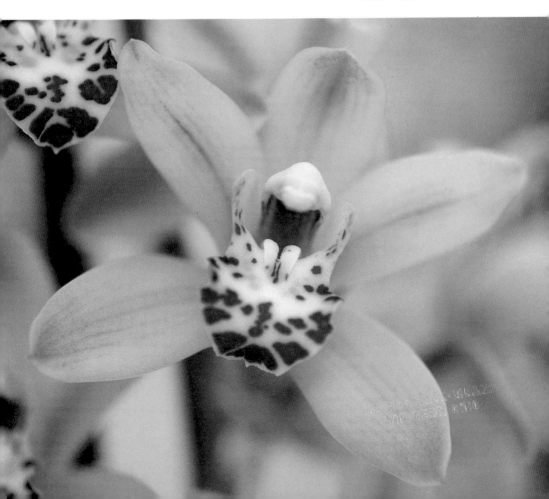

Contents

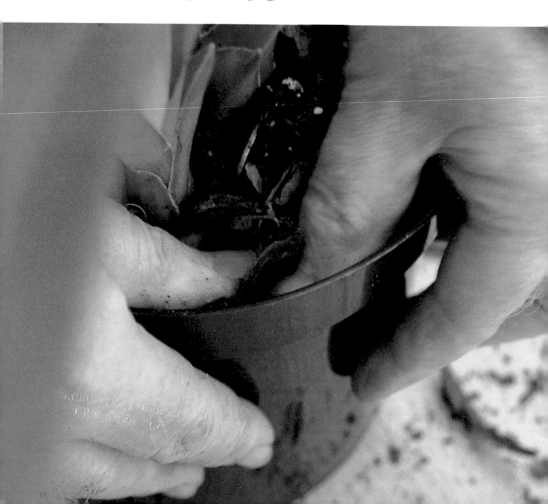

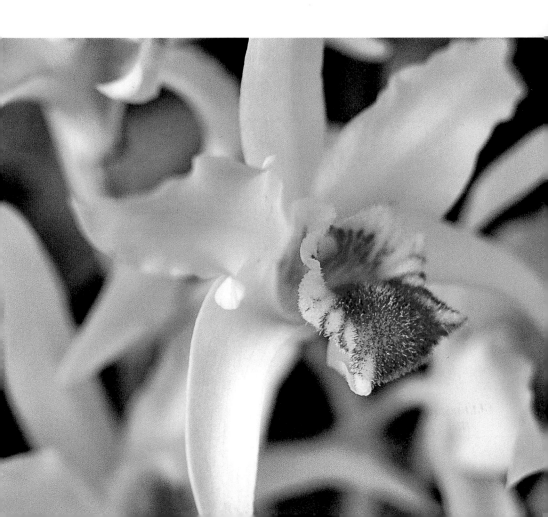

Introduction

Many plants have their devotees, but few give rise to such passion as orchids. Why is it that people become obsessed? Their beauty, strangeness and mystique must all play a part but perhaps most of all, their sheer variety appeals. If you like large, brightly coloured flowers, what is more flamboyant than a *Cattleya* hybrid? If you prefer purity of form and colour, nothing can surpass *Angraecum* and *Aerangis*. On the other hand, if your taste runs to the bizarre, you are spoilt for choice; they come in all sizes from the huge flowers of *Stanhopea* to the small flowers of many *Bulbophyllum* species. Orchids also provide scented flowers; many are strongly scented, both during the day and in the evening. Furthermore, orchid growing is an all-year-round hobby – there is always something in flower.

People come to love orchids in many ways. Sometimes they visit a flower show and are captivated by an orchid display; in other cases they may receive one as a gift. But probably the most common way is by buying a plant in flower from a garden centre. If that does well, they may buy another and when the plants stop flowering, they will need to know how to bring them into flower again. This will lead them to buy a book or join an orchid society, and by that time, the orchid owner is hooked.

Most people start with a general collection, acquiring any plants they can. But often, possibly for reasons of space, they start to specialize in a particular kind of orchid that grows well in the conditions they have on offer, perhaps African orchids, scented orchids, miniature orchids or a genus such as *Phalaenopsis*. Many growers have a well-developed collector's instinct, and try to amass as many of a particular genus or group as possible, but others just enjoy the beauty of their plants – and usually in a warm, pleasant environment rather than a wet and windswept garden.

Orchids have been cultivated in China for as long as 3,000 years but, as far as we know, the first tropical orchid to be grown in Europe was the South and Central American species *Brassavola nodosa*, in the late 17th century. In Britain, orchids first appeared in cultivation in the 18th century. William Aiton, Superintendent of the famous Kew Gardens, produced *Hortus Kewensis*, a three-volume catalogue of plants growing in Kew Gardens. This was first published in 1789 and lists 15 species of exotic orchid, while the second edition, published in 1813, includes no less than 70 species.

Initially, growers had little success in keeping these orchids alive. Because they were tropical plants they were grown in stove houses, where the atmosphere was hot but dry. No one knew that many came from high altitudes and required cool, moist conditions. Gradually, however, often by trial and error, gardeners came to realize that not all tropical orchids needed high temperatures, but almost all did need a good level of humidity and plenty of ventilation, and before long some large collections were built up. It must be remembered, too, that before the days of air travel, orchids had to undertake long sea voyages to reach European shores and many would already be in poor condition by the time they reached the boat.

Nowadays, collecting orchids in the wild is, or is supposed to be, strictly controlled and almost all cultivated orchids are grown from seed or produced by meristem culture. Apart from preserving wild stock, these plants are in fact much better suited to greenhouse or windowsill cultivation.

Now that their needs are understood, it is a myth that orchids are difficult to grow. A few may be, but most are not and in fact they can be surprisingly difficult to kill. No one can hope to grow all varieties of orchids equally well, but by observing a few simple rules the majority are no more difficult than any other houseplant. It is another myth that they are expensive. Again, some are and wildly inflated prices for a particularly rare or desirable variety help to perpetuate this myth. However, mass production has brought the prices of popular varieties within reach of everyone, making orchids an affordable and immensely enjoyable hobby for all.

Brassavola nodosa was the first tropical orchid to be grown in Britain.

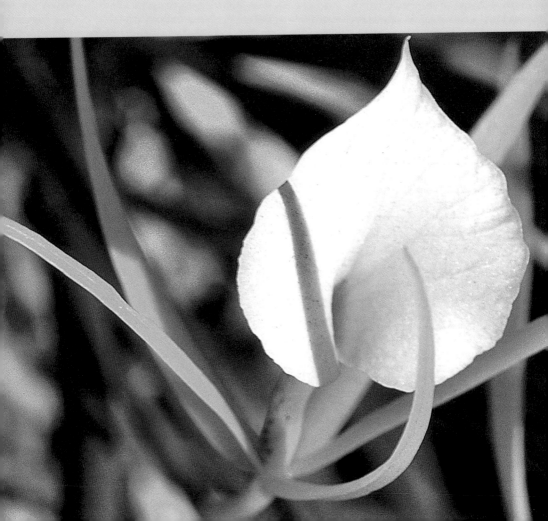

The orchid family, Orchidaceae, is probably the largest family of flowering plants in the world; with over 20,000 species in over 700 genera, its only possible rival is the daisy family, Compositae. Many orchid genera contain only one species but others are very large, for example *Bulbophyllum*, *Dendrobium*, *Epidendrum* and *Pleurothallis* are each thought to contain over 1,000 species. This may seem strange as orchids are often considered to be rare plants, and indeed many are confined to limited areas and specific habitats and consequently are at great risk from destruction of these habitats. Even common orchids tend to be local in their occurrence and do not dominate the vegetation in the way that certain other plants do.

The orchid family

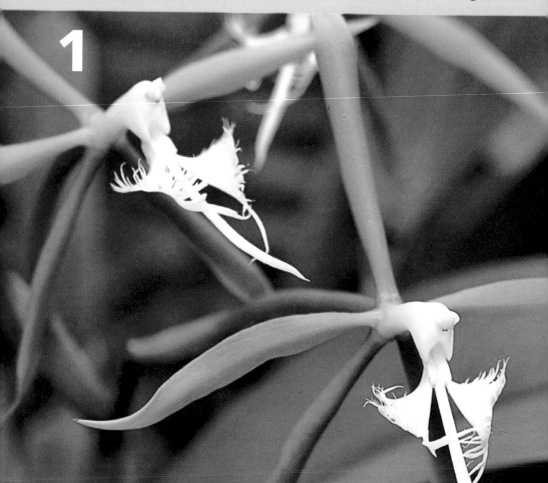

1

The orchid family

What is an orchid?

Why is an orchid an orchid – what are the distinctive features? Orchids are related to plants such as lilies. Like lilies, orchid flowers have three sepals and three petals but one of the petals, known as the lip or labellum, is always modified in some way. Often it is larger than the other petals and of a different shape or colour, sometimes marked with lines and blotches. In some orchids, for example *Cyrtorchis*, the lip is similar in appearance to the other petals but it carries a nectar-bearing spur at the base. Another distinctive feature is the reproductive parts of an orchid flower. The stamens, style and stigma (see page 46) are joined together to form a structure called the column, usually easily seen in the centre of the flower. In other plants, these structures are separate. Also, orchid pollen, instead of being loose as in most other plants, is joined into masses called pollinia.

Where orchids grow

Orchids can be found on every continent except Antarctica; some even grow inside the Arctic Circle. Between half and three-quarters of orchids are epiphytic, which means that they grow on other plants; the rest, including all native European species, are terrestrial, which means they grow on the ground. Epiphytes do not take any nutrients from their host – they simply use the host plant as a support or platform. It seems probable that orchids took to the trees to be nearer the light; the floor of a tropical forest is very dark and while some species became adapted to cope with these conditions, others moved upwards. It is easy to see how the habit

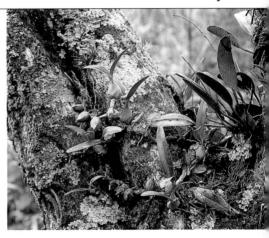

Epiphytic orchids in the wild.

developed: in the tropics, certain species that usually grow in leaf litter on the forest floor may sometimes be seen growing low down on tree trunks or in the forks of trees.

Orchids, of course, are not the only kind of epiphytic plant – in South American forests, bromeliads (often grown as air plants) are an important part of the epiphytic flora, and epiphytic ferns can be found all over the world. Some orchids grow on rocks and are known as lithophytes, but few species are consistently lithophytic. In the wild it is not uncommon to see a certain type of orchid growing on a tree, and nearby the same species flourishing on a rock. Terrestrial orchids may also grow on rocks on occasions, although in this case the roots or tubers are usually embedded in a layer of moss or humus rather than directly attached to the rock.

Epiphytic orchids

Most orchid species and the hybrids derived from them are tropical epiphytes. These plants have become adapted to their lifestyle in several ways, notably in their roots. Many have thick roots that fulfil a double function; as well as anchoring the plant to the branch or rock, the roots are surrounded by layers of dead cells called the velamen, which

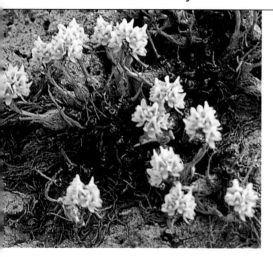

Polystachya brassii growing on a rock; it can also grow on trees.

readily absorb any available moisture. Even in tropical rainforests there is usually a dry season and in many places where orchids grow, the dry season can be quite severe. So epiphytic orchids are adapted in various ways to enable them to survive a period of drought, including their thick, leathery leaves that prevent moisture loss and their swollen stem bases, known as pseudobulbs, which also help conserve moisture.

How epiphytic orchids grow

Epiphytic orchids have two basic growth patterns: they may be monopodial or sympodial.

Monopodial These orchids have a leafy stem that grows continuously from the top although it may branch, usually at the base. This does not necessarily mean that these are tall plants; in many the amount of annual growth is very small and they remain compact. The flowers develop along the stems, usually in the leaf axils, and roots can also arise along the stem as well as at the base of the plant. After the resting season, growth resumes at the top of the stem. Monopodial orchids include vandas, phalaenopsis and angraecums.

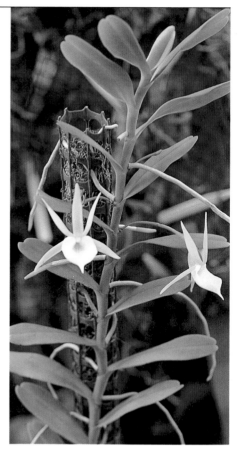

Angraecum birrimense is a monopodial or vandoid orchid.

Sympodial Sympodial orchids have a creeping rhizome (a horizontal stem growing either on or below the ground) with one or more new shoots arising

A new shoot grows from last year's pseudobulbs.

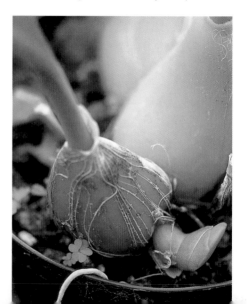

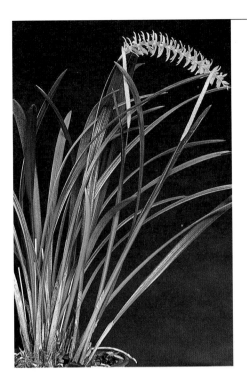

Slender pseudobulbs of *Dendrochilum javierense*.

from it each year. The flower spike often grows from the end of the stem, although it may arise at the base of the plant, beside the leafy growth. Most, but not all, sympodial orchids have pseudo-bulbs (swollen stem bases) which vary greatly in shape, size and arrangement. They may be large or small, round, ovoid, spindle-shaped or cane-like and may be set well apart on the creeping rhizome,

Ridged, conical pseudobulbs set close together.

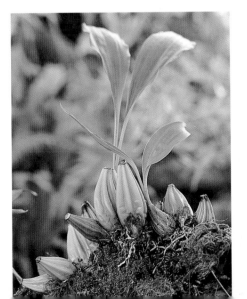

form clumps or grow from the previous year's pseudobulb and form a chain. Whatever the shape, pseudobulbs remain on the plant for several years, even after the leaves have been shed, and seem to have a storage function.

Terrestrial orchids

Terrestrial orchids also have different growth patterns. Some have creeping stems on or just below ground level with roots and clusters of leaves growing from them which may last for one or more years. The jewel orchids have this type of growth. Most terrestrial orchids have some sort of underground storage organ that keeps the plant alive while it is dormant. The dormant, or resting, season is winter in cool temperate climates, the hot dry summer in parts of the world with a Mediterranean-type climate, or the dry season in the tropics. The storage organs may be fleshy roots,,

Dactylorhiza foliosa, the Madeira orchid, adds rich colour to a garden.

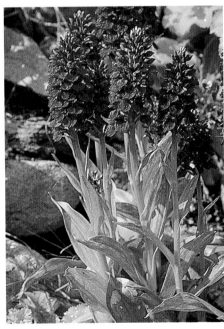

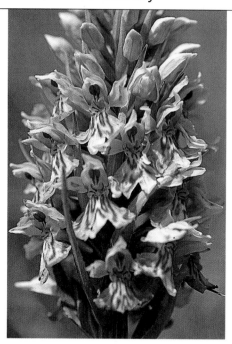

The Common Spotted Orchid, *Dactylorhiza fuchsii*, is widespread in Europe.

corms, tubers or pseudobulbs that are often partly above ground. Corms and pseudobulbs persist for several years, sometimes forming long chains, but tubers and fleshy roots are usually renewed each year.

Orchids in the wild

While it is never possible to reproduce exactly the conditions in which orchids grow in the wild, it helps to know what these conditions are. For example, as we have seen, in the early days of orchid growing most imported species died because they were grown in a hot, dry atmosphere. Once it was known that many orchids, although they came from the tropics, are high-altitude plants used to relatively cool, moist conditions, things began to improve.

Epiphytic orchids in the wild

Epiphytic orchids are naturally forest or woodland plants. This is why so many orchids are endangered, as all over the world, tropical forest and woodland is being felled for fuel or to clear land for farming. It follows that most are shade-loving plants – few like full exposure to sunlight. Some grow in surprisingly dark conditions, such as low down on tree trunks in dense forest, and even those that grow high up in the branches get some shade from the leafy canopy. In the wild, few orchids grow where the dry season is long and severe but almost all have to survive some period of relatively adverse conditions. So in cultivation almost all benefit from a rest when they are kept cooler and drier than when in active growth, and in fact many will not flower without such a rest. As a general rule, the thicker an orchid's roots, the less water it needs when not in active growth. Most orchids with fine roots, particularly those without pseudobulbs, are forest plants used to a short dry season.

Terrestrial orchids in the wild

Terrestrial orchids occur in a great range of habitats. The only common factor is that few, if any, can cope with competition from other plants. If grass is not kept short by grazing or controlled cutting, scrub develops and the orchids vanish.

In equatorial regions there are more epiphytic orchids than terrestrial but the further one moves from the equator, the higher the proportion of terrestrials. Few terrestrial orchids grow in the deep shade of the tropical forest floor but some do and this gives a clue to the conditions they like – warm, humid and shady. More can be found in open woodland, usually where the soil is poor and stony, but probably most species occur in grassland. Such plants do not take well to cultivation so they should only be attempted by the skilled grower, and in any case, most are difficult to obtain.

Orchid conservation

Many species of orchid have suffered greatly from over-collecting and some are even believed to be extinct in the wild. In an attempt to combat this, all orchids, both species and hybrids, are covered by the Convention on International Trade in Endangered Species (CITES). This means that orchid plants may not be brought or sent from one country to another without an import permit issued by the importing country and an export permit from the country of export. Free movement is, however, allowed within countries belonging to the European Union. A health certificate is also required. Furthermore, almost all countries have their own laws forbidding collection of wild orchids. Orchid seedlings in flasks (see page 48), however, are exempt from CITES regulations and do not need a health certificate.

Orchid names

Only a few orchids have a common name and even when they do, it tends to be a name for a group rather than for a particular species.
For example,
Miltoniopsis hybrids
are known as pansy orchids,
Phalaenopsis
are known as moth orchids and
Coryanthes
are known as bucket orchids.

So even a beginner has to become familiar with the botanical names.

Plant names are covered by a Code of Nomenclature. Orchid species, like other plants, have two names.

The first name, **the generic name**, begins with a capital letter and is given to all plants in the same genus, for example *Angraecum*.
The second name is **the specific name** and belongs to one species, for example *eburneum*, which is the specific name of the orchid *Angraecum eburneum*.
There may be, in addition, subspecies or varieties –
we can have
Angraecum eburneum subsp. *eburneum*;
Angraecum eburneum subsp. *giryamae* and
Angraecum eburneum subsp. *superbum*.
There is even
Angraecum eburneum subsp. *superbum* var. *longicalcar*.

The naming of hybrids is explained in Chapter 6.

Awards

Plants offered for sale may have letters after the name, such as FCC, AM or HCC. The first stands for First Class Certificate and is the highest award; AM is Award of Merit and is the next highest; HCC stands for Highly Commended Certificate. These awards are given by judging authorities such as the Royal Horticultural Society (RHS) and the American Orchid Society (AOS) – in these cases, the initials RHS or AOS should come after the award. Awards are an indication of quality and are given to a particular plant and not to the species or hybrid as a whole and so any awarded plant must have a cultivar name which begins with a capital letter and is enclosed in single quotation marks; for example, *Epidendrum revolutum* 'Burnham' AM/RHS and *Pleione* Shantung 'Ridgeway' AM/RHS..

Orchids can be grown in many places: in a greenhouse, on a windowsill, in a special case or under artificial lights, say, in a basement. In the tropics they can be grown in a shade house or in the garden. Orchids, like other plants, need water, light, nutrients and an adequate temperature if they are to thrive. If the grower can provide the right requirements, no matter where, the plants should be successful.

Where to grow orchids

2

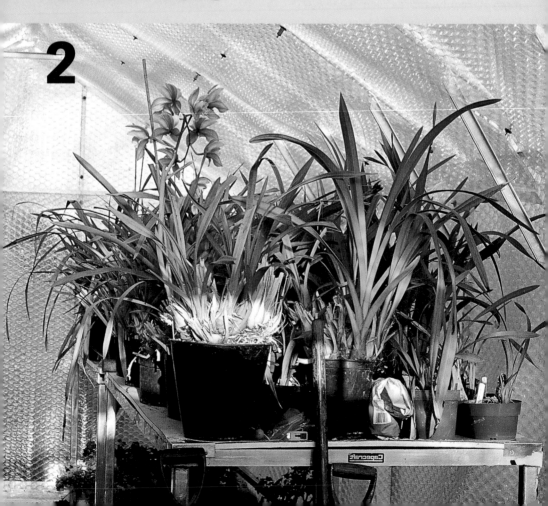

Where to grow orchids

Greenhouses

A greenhouse is probably the most popular place to grow orchids. Sometimes there will be an existing greenhouse in the garden, but often the new grower has to build one and in that case there are choices to be made. Greenhouses can have metal or wooden frames, have glass to the ground or solid walls at the base, and be glazed with glass or polycarbonate. Each type has its advantages and disadvantages. Wooden structures tend to look more attractive and it is easier to fix things like insulation and electrical appliances to the walls but they are more expensive to buy, require more maintenance and are more difficult to clean. Solid walls up to staging level are more heat-efficient but the lack of light low down means that plants cannot be grown under the staging.

A prospective purchaser should look at catalogues from a number of greenhouse suppliers, but the most important thing is to visit orchid houses and talk to growers to determine what is likely to suit best. Whatever type of greenhouse you choose, it is a good idea to buy the biggest you can afford and accommodate. The smaller the greenhouse, the greater is the surface area to volume ratio and the more difficult it is to maintain a stable temperature. Do not think that as you have only a few plants, you only need a small greenhouse – filling the space will be the least of your problems. Consider a minimum of 3 x 2.4m (10 x 8ft), and if possible have one that is 3.6m (12ft) wide, so that another block of staging can be fitted in the centre to give a more efficient use of space.

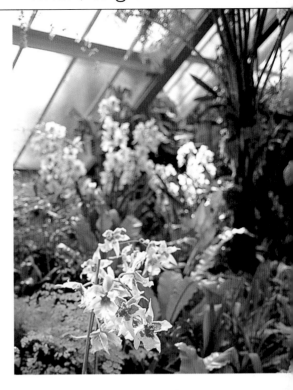

Orchids growing in a metal framed greenhouse

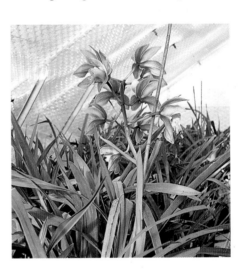

Cymbidiums in a greenhouse.

Siting a greenhouse

Siting a greenhouse is usually a matter for compromise. Ideally, it should not be overhung by large trees, the long axis should run east to west and it should be close enough to the house to have its own electrical and water supplies. But such a site is rarely found in a garden. Sometimes a lean-to greenhouse is the only option.

Greenhouse manufacturers advise that the corner posts should be set in concrete, but it is a good idea to have the whole greenhouse anchored in a concrete base. Apart from the extra strength – essential in exposed areas – a concrete base makes it more difficult for slugs, snails, mice and other such unwelcome visitors to enter.

Glazing materials and insulation

Glass is still the most widely used glazing material but polycarbonate sheeting has many advantages: it is lighter, virtually unbreakable and can be used as a double layer to give built-in insulation. However, it is still more expensive than glass. Other clear plastic materials are not suitable as they become cloudy and denatured after a few years. It is possible to have glass double glazing but this is very heavy and would probably require a specially designed building. Otherwise, glass greenhouses need some form of insulation to keep heating costs down. The most widely used is bubble polythene, which is attached to the inside of the greenhouse. It can be tacked to the frame of a wooden greenhouse; metal greenhouses have grooves in the frame and special plastic pegs are used to fix the lining. Bubble polythene is available in rolls in a choice of widths, together with the pegs and strong adhesive tape. It is available with large or small bubbles; the former is more effective. Unfortunately polythene has a limited life, up to about seven years; it then starts to break up and has to be replaced.

Heating methods

After deciding on the type of greenhouse to buy, the next step is to decide how to heat it. Again, each method has advantages and drawbacks. Electricity is the most widely used; it is usually the cheapest to install, is the cleanest and most convenient and offers the most control. The drawbacks are that it can be expensive to run, particularly in a large greenhouse, and of all the methods, it is the most likely to fail. The days of power cuts may be past but winter storms still take their toll.

In the early days of orchid growing, greenhouses had hot-water pipes running under the staging, heated by a solid-fuel boiler. Hot water pipes still offer a good form of heating, providing an even heat that does not give off fumes or dry out the air too much. These pipes come in two diameters, 10cm (4in) and 5cm (2in). The narrower pipes give a faster response but need an electric pump to circulate the water. Water in the larger pipes circulates by convection, and the pipes retain heat longer.

Oil-fired and gas-fired greenhouse boilers are available and although the initial cost may be higher, running costs should be lower than with electricity. As long as the boiler is gravity fed and does not require an electric pump, it will keep going even if the electric power supply fails and as hot-water pipes retain their heat for several hours, there is no sudden loss of temperature if something goes wrong. These boilers have controls but they are not as flexible as the control available with electrical heating.

If a greenhouse is very near or attached to a house, it is a good idea to heat it through the house central heating as long as the system is not set to switch off at night.

Back-up heating

Whatever method is used, it is almost certain to fail at some time and it is essential to have some other kind of heating in reserve, as a whole collection of orchids can be lost overnight. With gas- or oil-fired systems, electric fan-heaters can serve as a back-up. Otherwise, paraffin or bottled gas heaters can be kept for use in an emergency.

Shading

Few orchids enjoy strong light so some sort of shading is necessary in the summer months and this also helps to prevent overheating. The cheapest and easiest method of shading is to paint the glass white; special paints for this are available from most garden centres. These paints are water resistant, but are easily rubbed off. Shade cloth or lath blinds are also effective and are most efficient when fixed to the outside of the house and raised above the glass, but this is not too easy to arrange and is not practical in a windy area.

Ventilation

In the wild, epiphytic orchids grow in airy places and good air movement in a greenhouse leads to better growth and fewer problems with fungus. All greenhouses have vents in the roof and these can be automatically controlled so that the plants can be left for a day or more without the worry of overheating, or of sudden draughts should the weather change for the worse. Automatic vents are usually available from the greenhouse manufacturer as an optional extra. They do not need a supply of electricity; simple and effective kinds operate using bimetallic strips or oil-filled cylinders.

One or two fans are also beneficial in a greenhouse, ideally sited over a pathway so that the moving air does not blow directly on to the plants. Fan heaters are a good investment as they can be set to heat the greenhouse or merely to move the air about to provide ventilation without additional heat.

Humidity

Almost all orchids like high humidity and this can be difficult to achieve especially in summer when the air is warm and the greenhouse vents are open. The old-fashioned method of raising humidity is by 'damping down'; the floor and under staging is sprayed with water and as this evaporates, the humidity rises. This method can still be used today if a greenhouse has no electrical supply.

However, various kinds of automatic humidifiers are available. Ultrasonic nebulizers were originally designed to create a humid atmosphere for asthma sufferers and give off a cloud of what looks like cold steam, but they do not cover a very large area and so are better suited to small greenhouses. The drawbacks are that they are fairly bulky, and if they are working consistently, the water reservoir can run out in less than a day. Also the filters need to be cleaned regularly as they get clogged up. Other systems available run from the mains water supply and consist of a series of mist jets. Fine jets can be positioned wherever they are required and it is possible to control the level of relative humidity at which they come on. The advantage of these systems is that they keep going if the owner is away. The finer the jet the better, and they should not play directly on to plants in pots as soggy compost soon leads to rot. Mounted plants love it, however.

Lighting

Extra lighting is also an option in a greenhouse. It is useful for extending the day length and thus encouraging growth in winter, particularly when the winter day is very short. Ordinary white fluorescent tubes can be used. This subject is dealt with on page 22.

Alpine houses

Alpine houses differ from standard greenhouses in having extra vents near the base of the house; they are either completely unheated or just kept free of frost in winter. Quite a lot of orchids can be grown in a frost-free alpine house, including pleiones and Mediterranean species such as *Ophrys*. With many near-hardy orchids, it is not the cold but the wet that kills them in the open garden, so a cool alpine house can provide the perfect conditions. For more details, see Chapter 10.

Bletilla striata can be grown in the garden or in an alpine house.

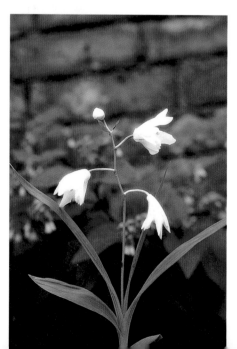

Staging

All greenhouses and alpine houses need staging and again there is a range of types available. Staging should not be too wide or it is difficult to reach plants at the back although tiered staging makes this easier. Slatted staging gives the free drainage that orchids like but the slats should not be set too far apart as a lot of orchids are grown in small pots.

Windowsills

Most people grow their first orchid with other houseplants on a windowsill and, if it is successful, they will acquire more orchids. At this stage, many people decide to invest in a greenhouse but others continue to grow large collections in the house, often very successfully. Temperature is seldom a problem here; the most difficult aspect is providing sufficient humidity without the walls and curtains sprouting green mould.

Kitchens and bathrooms are favoured places for indoor orchids as they tend to have higher humidity than other rooms, but orchids can be grown in any room that is warm enough. The usual solution is to have the pots sitting on trays containing a layer of moisture-retentive material, such as expanded clay pellets or perlag. This gives a humid atmosphere round the plants but the pots sit on the pellets, not in the water, thus preventing the soil from becoming waterlogged. It is always better to arrange orchids in groups rather than singly, as plants create their own humidity.

In the Northern Hemisphere, site plants close to an east- or west-facing window as a south-facing window is likely to be too hot in summer although

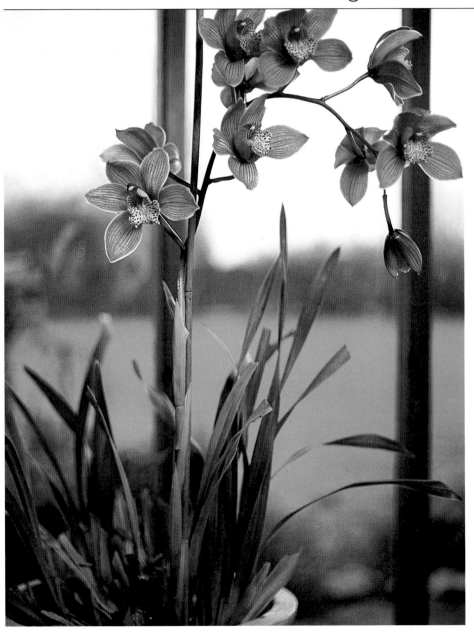

Cymbidium hybrids do well as house plants.

good in winter. Net curtains will help to screen the scorching effects of direct sun or plants can, of course, be placed on a table set back slightly from the window – a bay window is particularly suitable for this. It goes without saying that the window should not be draughty. Orchids should not be put on top of a radiator or a television set where they will get too hot and dry. For obvious reasons, miniature orchids are best suited for house culture. A list of suitable species is given below, although many others could well be successful.

Plants to grow on a windowsill

Aerangis fastuosa
Angraecum didieri and *rutenbergianum*
Brassavola nodosa
Cattleya intermedia and *skinneri*
Cattleya hybrids, particularly

'mini-cattleyas'
Coelogyne cristata and *nitida*
Cymbidium devonianum and
   floribundum
Cymbidium miniature hybrids
Dendrobium kingianum
Dendrobium nobile and hybrids
Encyclia cochleata and *vitellina*
Laelia anceps and *gouldiana*
Ludisia discolor
Masdevallia species and hybrids
Maxillaria tenuifolia
Paphiopedilum callosum
Phalaenopsis hybrids
Pleione species and hybrids
Stenoglottis species

Artificial lights

The practice of growing orchids under artificial lights seems to be more common in America than in Europe. It enables parts of a house such as a basement, cellar or loft to be used as a growing area. This has much to recommend it as the area is likely to be heated to some extent already and, being enclosed, it will tend to have a fairly high humidity. Growing orchids under lights gives the grower almost complete control over growing conditions. It is possible to have a day length of 12–16 hours all year round so that plants grow continuously, although this would be better for young stock than for mature flowering plants, where some seasonal variation is desirable.

It is possible to buy 'grow lights' specially formulated for optimum plant growth. However, the blue and red parts of the spectrum are the wavelengths mainly used in photosynthesis (the process by which green plants use light to produce energy) and these are supplied by white fluorescent tubes. Ordinary incandescent light bulbs give light in the red part of the spectrum, which helps to trigger flowering, and so a combination of the two kinds should give good results. Four 40-watt fluorescent tubes and four 8-watt incandescent bulbs would be a suitable arrangement. The lights are usually fixed on to a piece of wood that is suspended on chains from the ceiling, allowing them to be moved up and down. The lights should be 15–45cm (6–18in) above the leaves; obviously light-loving orchids such as *Cattleya* should be positioned near the lights and those that prefer more shade, such as *Phalaenopsis*, should be further away. Remember that lights also give off heat. In any enclosed area ventilation is essential, and fan heaters are most suitable for this.

Orchid cases

Orchid cases are direct descendants of the glass Wardian cases that were first used in the mid-19th century to improve survival rates of orchids and other plants which had to endure long sea voyages. In 1842, the English nursery firm Loddiges said that after they started using Wardian cases, the survival rate of imported plants rose from five per cent to ninety-five per cent.

As these cases obviously provided excellent growing conditions, they began to be used in other ways and in late Victorian times they became very fashionable. By this time, Wardian cases had changed from the original wooden glass-topped boxes to decorative structures, usually entirely of glass, often in elaborate shapes such as a miniature model of the Crystal Palace in South

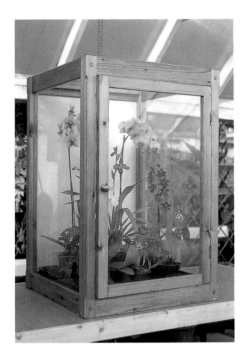

Orchid cases can make an attractive feature in a room.

London. Not many of these survive and those that do are collectors' pieces, but simpler cases are still used to grow orchids successfully and make a decorative feature in a living room. Heat, light and humidity can be controlled automatically in such cases.

A small orchid collection can be grown entirely in this way, and people with larger collections sometimes use them for difficult species that need carefully controlled conditions, as well as for their decorative effect. Few, if any, firms still make orchid cases, but they are still occasionally available second-hand. Otherwise, it is not too difficult to have one made; a number of firms could supply the necessary controls. A typical size is about 1.5m (5ft) high by 1.2m (4ft) wide and 60cm (24in) deep – these are the outside measurements; the growing area is slightly smaller. The floor of such cases usually consists of a waterproof tray with aggregate granules under which there is a heating cable set on a wooden base with a movable grill to control air flow. The wooden roof has vent holes but a small fan may also be necessary as good ventilation is essential. For a cabinet of this size, three 40-watt fluorescent tubes should be sufficient; they can be controlled by a time switch set to give 12–14 hours of light a day. Keep 2.5cm (1in) of water in the tray to keep the humidity high.

Plants to grow in an orchid case

Aerangis, most species
Angraecum, smaller species
Cattleya, small hybrids
Dendrobium bigibbum
Dendrobium hybrids
Dracula species
Ludisia discolor and other jewel orchids
Paphiopedilum, most species and
  hybrids
Phalaenopsis species and hybrids
Pleurothallis species

Shade houses

Shade houses are used for growing orchids in tropical and subtropical climates where the problem is one of too much heat and light, rather than cold. They are usually simple structures made from poles with a thatched or shade-cloth roof, often with shade-cloth or polythene curtains on the sides that catch the sun. They have the great advantage of being easy and cheap to extend when the need arises.

Given the right conditions, most orchids are no more difficult to grow than other plants. They can be grown in pots, in baskets or mounted on bark or tree fern slabs. Pots may be plastic or clay. Nowadays, plastic pots are more often used as they are cheaper, lighter and easier to clean and it is easier to get an orchid out when repotting as the roots do not cling so tightly to plastic as they do to clay. Terrestrial orchids, however, which are particularly sensitive to overwatering, do better in clay pots as the soil dries out much more quickly.

How to grow orchids

3

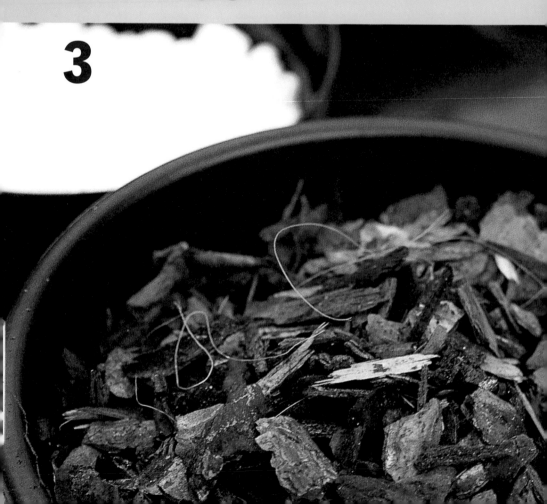

How to grow orchids

As growers become more involved in their hobby, they want to add all sorts of refinements, especially if they have a greenhouse. It is possible to grow orchids in a completely automated way, but this should not be at the expense of giving the plants personal attention. There is no substitute for the grower's eye. Automatic systems are useful, however, as they make it possible for the grower to go away without making complicated arrangements with neighbours to look after the plants.

Epiphytic orchids

Most epiphytic orchids can be grown in pots. It is often suggested that extra holes be drilled or burnt in pots to improve the drainage, but adding a layer of drainage material such as polystyrene chips in the bottom of the pot is just as effective. Baskets and rafts are useful where a plant has a creeping habit and keeps climbing out of a pot – cattleyas and many *Bulbophyllum* species behave like this.

Baskets

Baskets are essential for orchids such as stanhopeas where the flower spike actually grows downwards from the roots. Draculas have the same habit but as they are small plants with wiry flower spikes, a plastic mesh pot is often used. Baskets are also often used for orchids such as vandas with long, vigorous roots – in fact, vandas are sometimes grown in empty baskets with no compost at all. Wooden baskets can be bought but are very easy to make at home.

Mounts

Mounts are used for smaller plants that do not like to have their roots

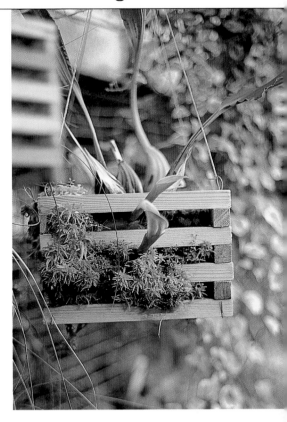

Many orchids do well in a wooden basket.

confined in pots, such as most species of *Mystacidium*, and for plants with long-spurred flowers, such as *Aerangis* species.

Mounts and rafts can be made of a variety of materials such as slabs of cork, fir or pine bark, pieces of tree fern or small branches. Pieces of cork bark are the most traditional. They can often be bought from a florist, but are becoming expensive; thick pine bark that has separated from the outside of a log of firewood, can be equally good. The bark should be at least 1cm (½in) thick or it will not last. Bore a hole at one end and fit a neat wire hook through it so that the mount with its plant can be hung up in a shaded, humid place.

When pieces of wood are used as mounts, people tend to have their own favourites – some swear by apple, others by gorse. Most orchids prefer a textured piece where the roots can make their

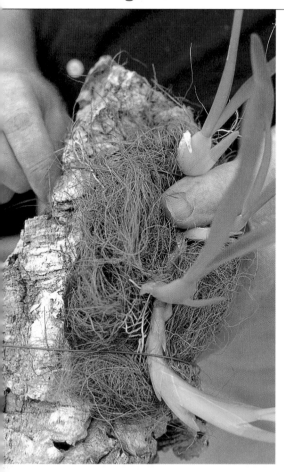

Mounted orchids must be firmly tied to the bark.

become firmly attached and no longer needs it. Thin strips cut from tights or stockings are also good, but raffia rots too quickly. Mounted orchids need higher humidity than plants in pots because they have no compost from which to draw moisture, so it is helpful to place a small piece of moss behind the plant to keep it moist until it is established.

Potting composts

Bark mixes While orchids can be grown in all sorts of media, including coir, sphagnum moss and perlite, the most frequently used composts are based on chopped bark. Special orchid bark must be used. The partly composted bark that is sold as a mulch in garden centres is not suitable. Orchid bark is available in three grades. Fine grade is used for seedlings and often as part of other mixes; medium or standard grade is used for most flowering-size orchids and coarse grade is used for large, thick-rooted plants. It is advisable to wash or sieve the bark before using it to get rid of the powdery dust that always seems to be present to some extent. Bark can be used on its own but composts are usually a mixture of bark, perlag or super-coarse perlite, and horticultural grade charcoal; they can be bought ready mixed or the grower can mix up his own.

way into crevices, but a few species pre-fer smooth bark such as birch, or even a plain wood surface. Driftwood looks attractive, but if it comes from the sea, all the salt must be washed or weathered out. When an orchid outgrows its mount, the whole arrangement can be tied on to a larger mount.

When mounting a plant, fasten it on firmly – if the roots can move about, they are less likely to adhere to the bark. Various materials are used to tie orchids to their mounts. Fishing line is popular as it is very unobtrusive, but it can be diffi-cult to handle and there is always the possibility of it cutting into stems or roots as they grow thicker. String is a good alternative; it has a limited life but usually by the time it has rotted, the orchid has

Every 'recipe' seems to use these ingredients in slightly different propor-tions and it is not necessary to be too exact. A good mixture is six parts of bark to one part of coarse perlite and one part of charcoal. Sometimes coarse peat or chopped sphagnum moss is included, but this makes the mixture very water retentive, so care must be taken not to overwater.

For orchids past the seedling stage, mixes based on medium bark are most suitable, unless the roots are very fine. Whether coarse or fine, there should be free, open drainage and as soon as the compost shows signs of starting to decompose, the plant should be repotted.

Almost all orchid houses become populated with ferns; under the staging, they are attractive and help to keep up humidity but do not let them grow in orchid pots as fern roots break down bark and the compost soon becomes a soggy mess. Moss is also undesirable in a pot (although acceptable, within reason, on a mount) as it tends to draw all the moisture from the compost.

Rockwool This is becoming increasingly popular as a potting mix. It is spun from molten volcanic rock, rather like fibreglass, and as it does not decompose like an organic mix, repotting should be necessary only when a plant outgrows its pot. Repotting from and into rockwool causes less disturbance than with bark-based mixes as the roots do not need to have all the old mixture shaken off.

Rockwool can be bought on its own in water-repellent and water-absorbent forms, but it is easier to buy it ready mixed as a complete potting mixture. Some mixtures also contain perlite. If perlite is not already included, add 30-50 per cent to the mixture to improve aeration. This will make the potting mix dry out quickly, so be vigilant with watering and do not have orchids growing in rockwool on the same bench as orchids growing in a bark mixture; the watering requirements are too different. If you wish to use both media, keep the plants in separate groups to avoid over- or underwatering. Rockwool supplies no nutrients at all so add fertilizer regularly.

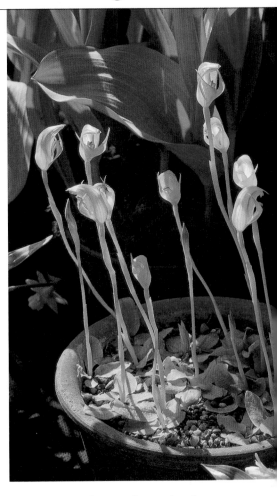

Pterostylis curta is a popular species of terrestrial orchid.

Terrestrial orchids

Although less common in collections than epiphytes, some terrestrial orchids are widely cultivated, such as *Calanthe* and *Disa* hybrids which are becoming steadily more popular.

Growers who specialize in terrestrial orchids say that they are no more difficult than epiphytes, but not everyone agrees. An epiphytic orchid is visible all year round and it is usually easy to see if there is something wrong, while most terrestrials disappear completely underground when they are dormant. When growing terrestrial orchids it is essential to follow the plant's natural rhythm. A few species are evergreen but most are deciduous and usually the leaves start to turn yellow and die back after flowering; this is a signal that the plant is ready to go into its resting period and should be kept dry.

Sprinkle some water on the surface every week or so during the dormant period or the tubers will shrivel, but don't start watering properly until the new shoots have grown 2.5cm (1in) above ground. Then carefully apply the water using a can with a fine spout – if any gets on to the new growth it is likely to turn black.

If you use clay pots to grow terrestrial orchids, plunge them in sand; during dormancy, keep the sand damp to provide enough moisture to stop roots or tubers from shrivelling, but not enough to make them rot.

Potting composts for terrestrial orchids

Various composts are recommended for terrestrial orchids but the exact ingredients are less important than the fact that they must be free draining – even species that grow in bogs and marshes in the wild will die if kept constantly wet in cultivation. Overwatering is the most common cause of death of terrestrial orchids; it is a useful rule to allow the compost to dry out before watering again. More or less the same ingredients occur in the suggested compost mixes, so obviously a fair bit of flexibility is possible. Disas, however, are a special case; their requirements are given later (see page 64).

Mix 1
1 part peat or peat substitute
1 part sterile loam
1 part coarse sand

Mix 2
2 parts sphagnum moss peat
1 part coarse sand
1 part perlite

Mix 3
3 parts sterile loam
3 parts coarse sand or grit
2 parts sieved beech or oak leaf mould
1 part fine orchid bark

Mix 4
3 parts fibrous peat
2 parts coarse perlite
2 parts coarse grit
1 part horticultural grade charcoal

Temperature

Orchids are classified by the temperatures that they require to grow successfully and are divided into warm, intermediate and cool. Warm-growing orchids require a night-time minimum temperature of 18°C (65°F) and, ideally, a daytime maximum of 27°C (80°F). Intermediate orchids need a night-time minimum of 13–15° (55–60°F) and an ideal maximum of 27°C (80°F). Cool-growing orchids require a minimum of about 10°C (50°F) with a maximum of 21°C (70°F). For any group, if the temperature occasionally falls a few degrees below the minimum it is unlikely to do harm, but it must be remembered that the cooler it is, the drier the plants should be kept. There should be a daytime rise in temperature of at least 5°C (10°F) although a short spell without this should not be harmful – it can be difficult to get much rise in a cold, dull spell in winter.

Maximum temperature is often more difficult to control than minimum and most orchids suffer in temperatures of over 35°C (95°F); it is best not to let it rise much over 30°C (86°F). At these high temperatures, high humidity is very important and frequent damping down and spraying also has a cooling effect.

With electrical heating systems, it is possible to control temperature very accurately, less so with systems which depend on hot-water pipes, which seem to have a particular range at which they run best. For example, in our greenhouse, a system using 10cm (4in) hot-water pipes heated by a gravity-fed, oil-fired boiler naturally gave intermediate conditions.

A large orchid house may be divided into cool, intermediate and warm sections, but this is rarely possible for the amateur grower, who must choose their temperature. The widest range of orchids can be grown in an intermediate house. All greenhouses, whatever their basic temperature, have warmer and cooler spots and the observant grower soon finds these out. By careful positioning and a bit of trial and error, you may be able to grow a wider range of plants than you expect.

Watering

Watering is the aspect of orchid growing that causes the most worry to beginners and experienced growers alike. The old maxim applies here: 'When in doubt, don't'. Far more orchids die from over-watering than underwatering. It is impossible to lay down any hard and fast rules as to when to water because so many variables apply – temperature, ventilation, pot size, compost and the state of growth of the plant are some of the more obvious ones. A plant in new compost needs more water than one in a

compost that has started to break down and is less well aerated; likewise a plant in active growth uses more water than one that is resting. Small pots dry out more quickly than large ones; and mounted plants need to be watered – or at least sprayed – more frequently than plants in pots.

In winter, once a week or even once a fortnight may be enough for orchids in pots yet in summer they may require watering at least twice a week, perhaps every other day in a hot spell.

Water quality

There is no doubt about the importance of water quality. Epiphytic orchids are adapted to take in almost pure rainwater with very low levels of dissolved salts and nutrients. So water with a high proportion of mineral salts is not suitable for orchids. Many growers in areas where the mains water has a high percentage of dissolved salts use rainwater for watering; others use reverse osmosis units which are said to remove up to 98 per cent of dissolved salts. Hard water does not seem to be too harmful but an unsightly deposit of calcium salts builds up on leaves over time and can block the pores through which gas exchange takes place. If the water is highly chlorinated, leave it to stand overnight to remove most of the chlorine.

Water temperature

Whatever the source and quality of the water, it is important that it should be at air temperature rather than used straight from the mains. Watering with cold water causes black spots and blotching on leaves, which is unsightly in itself and may lead to fungal infection and bud drop. Sophisticated equipment is available, but it is simpler to have a water tank or drum in the greenhouse. Fill the tank each evening, allow it to stand overnight to warm up, then use the water the following day and refill the tank after you have finished. This system also helps to get rid of any excess chlorine in the water.

Watering cans are perfectly good for small collections of plants, but it is possible to rig up a pump and hose to take the hard work out of watering large collections. Use a submersible pump of the kind sold for fountains in ornamental ponds and connect it to a hose and watering lance. Place the pump in your water tank in the greenhouse so that it pumps the warmed water through the hose. Refill the tank from the mains after watering.

Feeding

Orchids have evolved to have low fertilizer requirements. In the wild, epiphytic orchids depend on minerals arising from the breakdown of bark, the occasional bird dropping and the very low amounts that have dissolved in rainwater, and almost all terrestrial orchids grow in areas with poor soil of low nutritional value. So any fertilizer must be applied in very dilute form. It is possible to buy fertilizers specially formulated for orchids and startling claims are made for many of these. However, ordinary houseplant fertilizers can be used as long as they are given at only a quarter to a half of the recommended strength.

Over time, bark is broken down by bacteria and these use up nitrogen. So orchids grown in bark-based composts need a high-nitrogen fertilizer. The source of the nitrogen should be nitrates, not urea, so check the composition given on the packet. Growers vary in how often they apply fertilizers; some go on the 'weakly, weekly' principle while others use a weak fertilizer solution for three waterings out of four. Whatever system is used and whatever the compost, it is important to flush the pots regularly with plain water to prevent any build-up of salts. Blackened root tips and black leaf tips are signs of too much fertilizer.

Types of fertilizer

The main elements supplied by a fertilizer are nitrogen, phosphorus and potassium and the composition is usually expressed in numbers shown on the packet – for example, 30:30:30 indicates a fertilizer with equal amounts of the three major nutrients. A high-nitrogen fertilizer will be shown as 30:10:10, while 10:10:30 indicates one that is high in potassium. Many growers use a high-nitrogen fertilizer in spring and early summer to promote growth, and change to a high-potassium mixture in late summer and autumn to give the next season's flowering a boost. One element that does not usually appear in fertilizers is calcium. In hard-water areas this is never in short supply but in soft-water areas, application of a weak solution of calcium nitrate is beneficial. Frequency of fertilizing should be reduced or even stopped altogether when orchids are not in active growth, which usually means in winter.

Light and shade

Orchids are often considered to be plants with high light requirements but few people who have not seen them growing in the wild realize in what deep shade some species grow. A few grow low down on tree trunks in dense forests, where a light meter gives no reading at all. More species grow higher up in the trees, usually on the larger branches, where there is a little more light, but very few grow right up in the canopy. Among the epiphytes, it is only really those that grow on rocks rather than trees that are used to more intense light. Even the terrestrial orchids that grow in the open, in bogs and grassland, often get some shade from grass.

Greenhouse variations

All greenhouses will have one area that is more shaded than another. If the greenhouse is aligned east to west, the staging running along the south side will be much brighter than that on the north side, which may be further shaded if there are plants hanging in the middle of the greenhouse. Orchids that like heavy shade can be hung below the staging, and so it is possible to accommodate most preferences.

It is not hard to tell by appearances if a plant is getting the right amount of light. If the shade is too heavy, it will have dark green and luxuriant foliage but may not flower, while if it is getting too much light it may flower well but have small, yellowish leaves.

Repotting

Repotting is necessary in three circumstances:

1
If a plant is obviously outgrowing its pot, then it should be moved to a larger pot with fresh compost. This is best done just as new roots are starting to develop; if they are too long, they are easily broken.

2
If the compost has broken down and has become denatured and soggy the plant should be repotted as soon as possible. If many of the roots have died, it can be repotted into the same size of pot or even a smaller one.

3
If a plant just seems to be sitting still, without making growth, then fresh compost often seems to give it a boost even though the original compost has retained its structure.

Sometimes even with plastic pots, roots cling to the inside of the pot and are difficult to detach without damage. In this case, soak the pot with its plant in a bucket of water for half an hour and usually the roots then come away quite easily. In all cases, dead roots should be cut away; they will be brown and feel soft when pressed lightly. Dead pseudo-bulbs can be removed at the same time. Do not be tempted to use too large a pot for repotting: an orchid should always be put into a pot which is only just big enough to accommodate its root system.

Well-grown orchids are, by and large, healthy plants but they can fall victim to any of the usual greenhouse pests, most of which also occur on houseplants. As in most things, prevention is better than cure and while it may be impossible to avoid an attack completely, the vigilant grower should be able to prevent a severe infestation. One simple rule is to keep the greenhouse as clean as possible and remove dead flowers and leaves regularly. While some pests, such as aphids, enter a greenhouse through open vents, most are introduced on other plants. Any new plant should be examined carefully before being introduced to a collection. Ideally, it should first go into a quarantine area but this is often not practical.

Pests and diseases

4

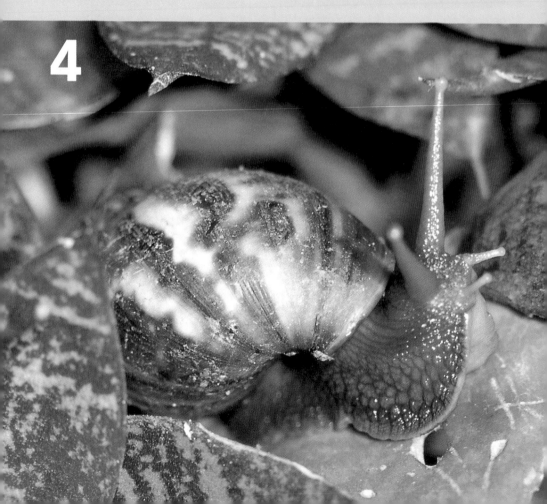

Pests and diseases

Controlling pests

Pests can be roughly divided into those that spend most of their life cycle on a plant, such as scale insects and red spider mite, and those that roam around seeking what they may devour, such as slugs, snails and woodlice. The latter group, although in general less serious, are often more difficult to deal with.

Biological control

Most greenhouse pests are themselves attacked by some kind of predator and these can sometimes be used by the grower to kill the pests. The big advantage of biological control is that it is very specific and only the pest is affected, not other insects which may be harmless or even beneficial. The main disadvantage is that the pests are never completely wiped out – it is not in the interest of a predator to kill off its food source entirely. A low level of infestation may not matter if the plants are grown purely for pleasure, but a professional grower cannot sell or show plants with damaged leaves. If biological control is being used it is not possible to use chemical methods at the same time. Several firms, which advertise in horticul-tural magazines, will supply the parasites and predators that are necessary.

Chemical control

As well as biological control, pests can also be controlled with chemical pesticides. Pesticides are either systemic or contact in their action. Systemic pesticides are taken up inside the plant and kill only pests that feed on that plant; other insects are unaffected. Contact pesticides are applied to the foliage of the plant; they are unselective and kill any pest that they touch but those that lurk in leaf axils, for example, may escape unharmed.

It might, then, seem obvious that systemic pesticides are preferable but they do not work in all cases. Scale insects, for example, do not take in enough plant sap to kill them.

All garden centres carry a good selection of pesticides. If you choose to use them, follow the instructions on the packet exactly, including the safety instructions. It goes without saying that you should always make sure that a chemical is recommended against the pest in question.

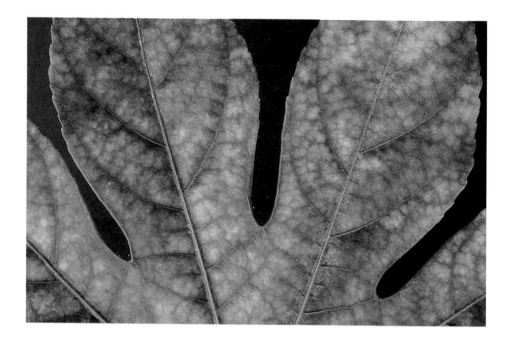

Spider mites

Red spider mite and false spider mite are probably the most serious pests of orchids because they are the most insidious. The creatures themselves are so small that they are difficult to see and usually the first warning is the silvery appearance of a plant's leaves, particularly the underside, which later turn brown. Red spider mite is often said to be more prevalent in dry conditions but it can still flourish when the humidity is high. In winter, when the day length is less than 12 hours, the mites may migrate to the frame of the greenhouse and hibernate within webs. So, if possible, wash the frame with dilute bleach at this time of year to help stop any build-up.

There is a predatory mite that provides a well-established means of biological control against spider mites. It should be introduced when red spider mite numbers are rising, that is in spring. It attacks all stages of the mite's life cycle – egg, nymph and adult. If chemical control is preferred, the insecticide has to be changed every few years as the mites develop resistance to chemicals. The eggs are immune to virtually all insecticides and so applications should be repeated after ten days by which time the eggs will have hatched.

False spider mite can also attack orchids and is susceptible to the same pesticides as red spider mite. It is particularly serious on pleiones, where it hides under the pseudobulbs and thus escapes contact with the pesticide. To deal with this problem, lift the pleiones, spray with the relevant pesticide and repot into fresh compost and clean pots.

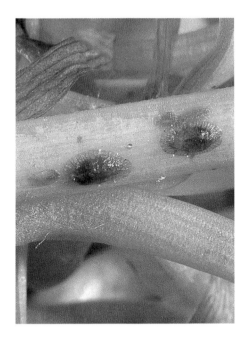 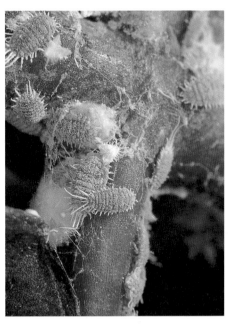

Scale insects

Several kinds of scale insects can affect orchids and all have a hardened, waxy shield which covers and protects the insect. They look rather like miniature limpets and, although small, are easy to see, unlike red spider mites. The waxy shield repels water and so insecticides carried in water are ineffective. Wiping the affected area with methylated spirit (known as rubbing alcohol in America) can clear a small infestation; a small brush or a cotton wool bud makes a good applicator. For larger infestations, white oil, malathion, dimethoate and diazinon are effective. Orchids often share a greenhouse with other plants, for example ferns, which are also susceptible to scale and these, too, must be checked. Adult scale insects do not move around, but newly hatched nymphs are mobile and can colonize a new area.

Mealy bugs

These insects belong to the same family as scale insects and are easily seen as they are covered by a white, waxy coating. They can be controlled by the same insecticides as scale insects, but biological control is also an option: a species of ladybird is available which is an effective predator but it needs a relatively high and stable temperature to succeed, around 21°C (70°F)

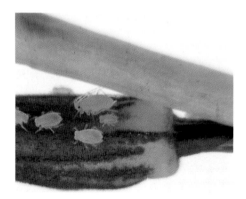

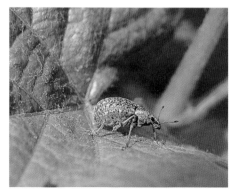

Aphids

All gardeners are familiar with aphids; greenfly and blackfly are facts of horticultural life. Although orchids are less susceptible than many plants, aphids are attracted by new growth and particularly by flower buds. Both young leaves and flowers can become badly distorted but the most serious aspect of aphid infestation is that they are important carriers of viruses. Most insecticides kill aphids but it should be possible to spot them when there are only a few, when they can easily be wiped off. However, they multiply quickly so the grower must be vigilant.

Vine weevils

Vine weevils, which seem to be on the increase, cause damage in two ways. The adults eat circular holes in leaves and the grubs, which are white with a brown head and are about 8mm (⅜in) long, live below the soil surface and feed on roots and tubers. The damage caused by adults is unlikely to be fatal but it is unsightly and long lasting. It is the grubs, however, that pose the biggest risk. You are unlikely to find grubs in a bark-based compound and they would certainly not like rockwool, but terrestrial orchids growing in a peat-based compost could be at risk.

The grubs can be killed by the insecticide Sybol, but biological control is also possible in the form of a parasitic nematode (a type of eel worm), which attacks both adults and larvae. Adults can enter a greenhouse through open vents and one way of controlling them is to use an insectocutor, an electrical insect killer, although it will kill any flying insect that is attracted to light. Vine weevils are very cryptic and emerge only at night. It is said that if one goes into a greenhouse after dark, any vine weevils there can be traced by the sound of crunching jaws.

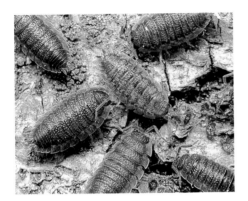

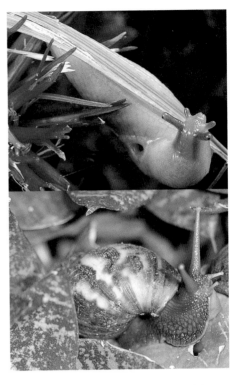

Woodlice

Woodlice feed mainly on decaying vegetable matter and many people believe that they do no harm to living plants, but they definitely eat the growing tips of orchid roots. They lurk under pots that are standing on a solid surface and you may occasionally find one in a pot when repotting. They probably do most damage to mounted orchids where they can hide under the plant or on the back of a mount, so it is always worth checking the backs of mounted plants from time to time. Woodlice are susceptible to almost any insecticide.

Slugs and snails

These are the bane of every gardener. If a greenhouse has a concrete base, that helps to prevent the entry of slugs but some always find their way inside where they live in and under pots and forage at night. The presence of chewed leaves and flower buds, and a trail of slime gives away their presence. They also climb and are just as likely to damage mounted plants. Slug pellets scattered around pots where slime trails are visible should be effective, and a saucer of beer on the greenhouse floor usually claims some victims. Frogs and toads, which often take up residence in a greenhouse, offer useful biological control. Another form is a nematode that lives off slugs, but there is unlikely to be a big enough population of slugs inside a greenhouse for this to be very practical.

Garlic snails

Garlic snails are tiny snails with a flat shell, about 5mm (¼in) in diameter, which are often found in orchid houses, being passed around between growers on pots and plants. They tend to live in the pots during the day and emerge in the evening. They do not seem to be affected by slug pellets, but reasonable control can be achieved by walking round the orchid house in the evening and crushing any that are seen. When crushed they smell of garlic, hence the name. At least growers in temperate climates are spared the depredations of the giant African snail, which grows to 15cm (6in) long and can demolish an orchid in a single day.

Preventing diseases

Not many fungal diseases are specific to orchids but leaf spotting caused by fungus is common. It usually occurs when a plant has been over-watered, particularly when the temperature is low and there is poor ventilation. Bacterial rot can set in if water lies for too long in leaf joints, and terrestrial orchids succumb very readily to stem rot if the compost is too wet while they are not in active growth.

Once again, prevention is better than cure. Watering should be carried out early enough in the day for leaves to be dry by nightfall when the temperature falls and the relative humidity rises. In the wild, of course, rain often falls at night but conditions there are very different from those in an enclosed glasshouse. In cases of fungal spotting, remove damaged leaves and spray the plant with a fungicide. With bacterial rot, it is usually too late to save the plant by the time it becomes evident; but in epiphytic orchids, if the stem and roots are firm, the plant may branch from lower down the stem. Any damaged tissue should be removed and the area treated with Physan or dusted with sulphur powder.

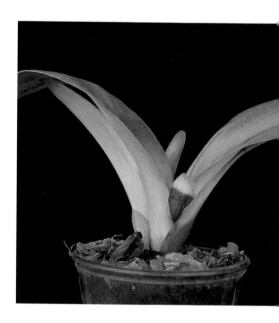

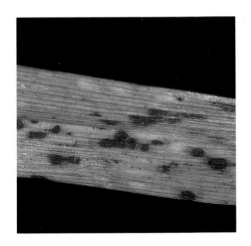

Viruses

Several viruses occur in orchids, the most common being cymbidium mosaic virus, which does not affect only cymbidiums although it is more common on them. The symptoms of viral infection are irregular, pale patches on young leaves that eventually turn brown or black, or sometimes yellow streaks on a leaf. At present there is no cure for viruses and an affected plant should be discarded before it affects others. Viruses can be transmitted from plant to plant in several ways; for example, by using a knife contaminated with sap from an affected plant to propagate an unaffected one, or by repotting into an affected pot. Obviously cleanliness is important; knives and scissors should be dipped in disinfectant before they are used, but it is not enough as one of the most common causes of virus spread is by sucking insects such as aphids.

Physiological damage

Not all marks found on an orchid's leaves are caused by infection or insect damage. Cold water on a leaf surface can cause black spotting, particularly on young leaves. This can be avoided by using water that is already at the temperature of the greenhouse and spraying only when the temperature is high.

Heat can cause damage as well as cold. Sunlight on a leaf can scorch it, particularly if the leaf is wet; unfortunately such marks are likely to remain on a plant for at least two years, until the leaf is finally shed. Yellow leaves may be caused by too much light or by mineral deficiencies – in the latter case the yellow is usually rather blotchy, whereas in the former the leaves will be an even yellow green. If you suspect a mineral deficiency, sprinkle a teaspoon of magnesium sulphate (Epsom salts) or iron sequestrene on the surface of the potting medium and water it in. Both are available in garden centres.

Blackening and dying of leaf tips is often the result of too strong a fertilizer or a build-up of salts in the compost. The best treatment is to repot the plant and make sure the circumstances do not arise again. Trim off the black tips; it does not usually spread but the plants look better for it.

Sometimes the new leaves on a plant appear as though they have been folded horizontally, as if to make a fan. This seems to be particularly prevalent in *Miltoniopsis* hybrids. This is caused by too dry a compost; if water is applied, the rest of the leaf should be smooth but the folded part remains, a permanent reminder of the owner's oversight.

All orchid growers want to increase
their plants at some time and
orchids, like other plants, can be
propagated either vegetatively
or from seed. For the average
grower, the former is by far the
most practical method.

Propagation

5

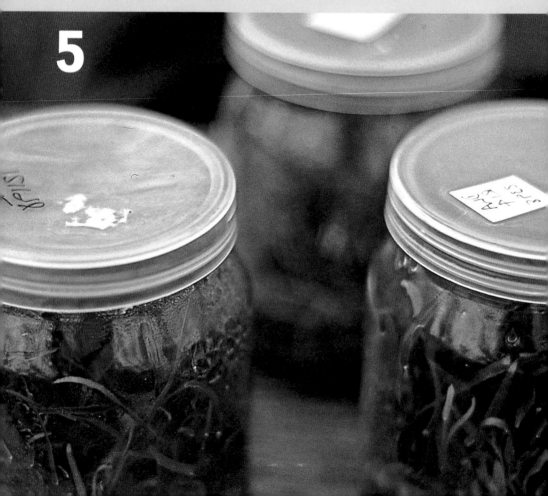

Propagation

Vegetative propagation

Vegetative propagation involves increasing a plant by division or from cuttings and results in two or more identical plants.

Sympodial orchids

Sympodial orchids are easily divided; they produce new growths every year and sometimes more or less divide themselves when the old, central growth dies. Division is best carried out when new roots are starting to develop on the new growths; if the roots are allowed to grow too long they can be difficult to fit into a pot and are more likely to break. Usually the leafy part of the growth and the roots develop together but in some plants the leafy growth may be fully formed before roots start to appear and then it is necessary to wait until the roots are growing before the plant is divided. The rhizome (creeping stem) is cut between two pseudobulbs or growths with a sharp, sterile knife or secateurs and the two (or more) parts are then potted up in the usual way. Do not be tempted to divide small plants, however; a division should have at least three pseudobulbs and preferably more.

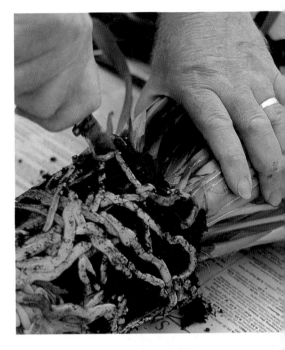

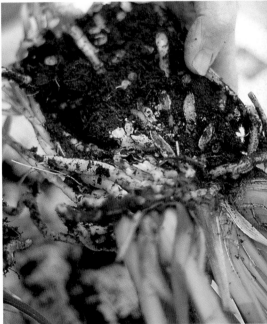

Above: The rhizome is cut with a sharp, sterile knife.

Below: The two parts of the plant are carefully eased apart.

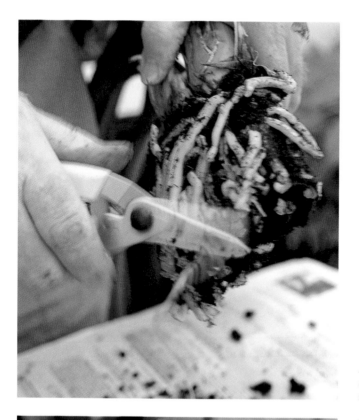

Above: The old roots are trimmed with sterile secateurs.

Below: The two halves of the original plant are now ready for potting.

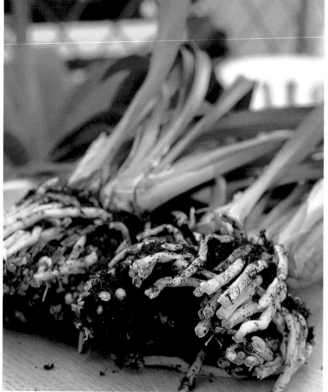

Back bulbs

Some orchids, such as cymbidiums, can be propagated from leafless back bulbs. Choose an old pseudobulb, cut it off at its base, and clean it up by removing any loose sheaths. Allow the cut edge to dry for a couple of days to lessen the risk of infection and then plant it to about a third of its height in perlite, grit or sharp sand and keep it cool and moist. A new shoot should appear within three months and once it has developed its own roots, which could take another two to three months, pot it up in standard compost. Another method is to put the back bulb in a polythene bag along with some damp sphagnum moss, seal the bag and hang it up in a warm, shady place. Leave it, as before, for two to three months until a shoot develops.

Monopodial orchids

Monopodial orchids are less easy to divide, but if the stems branch and the branches form their own roots, detach them and pot up as new plants. Vandas tend to develop long stems and become straggly. In almost all cases, the upper part of the stem has roots and if it is cut below some roots, the top part can be removed and treated as a new plant. The basal part will usually branch out and grow again.

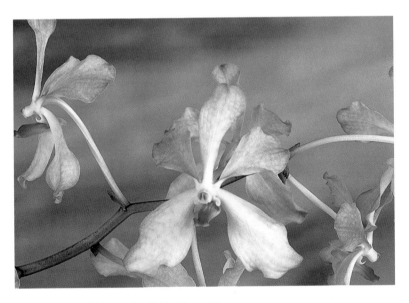

Monopodial orchids can be divided by cutting the stem between roots.

Keikis

Some orchids, both sympodial and monopodial, develop 'keikis' - this is a Hawaiian word meaning babies. These are small plants that grow from dormant buds on a pseudobulb or a flower spike. Many species of *Dendrobium* and *Epidendrum* develop keikis on their pseudobulbs, and some other orchids, such as *Phalaenopsis* and *Aeranthes*, occasionally produce them on the flower spikes. Once these little plants have developed a few short roots, they can be cut away with a sharp, sterile knife and potted up separately. The roots develop quickly and it is important to catch them before they grow too long and brittle.

Cuttings

Cuttings differ from divisions in that they do not have roots when they are removed from the parent plant. All gardeners are used to taking cuttings and there are a few orchids that will grow well from cuttings. Species of *Vanilla* can be increased in this way, as can some species of *Angraecum* such as *Angraecum distichum*. These cuttings produce roots much more readily in perlite than in bark and a heated propagator will speed things up greatly. Stems of many species of *Dendrobium* and *Epidendrum* can be cut into sections and either laid on a tray of damp moss or planted in perlite or grit. In this way, they will often produce new shoots provided a dormant bud is present. Any cuttings should be taken when the plants are growing actively, which will usually be in spring or summer.

Meristem propagation

Any method of vegetative propagation results in identical offspring, while propagation by seed does not. For this reason, a particular hybrid must be increased vegetatively rather than from seed, as seedlings are always variable. However, while taking cuttings and dividing plants are satisfactory methods for an amateur grower or small nursery, it takes a long time to build up a sizeable stock in this way. This is one reason why, in the past, particularly desirable forms of orchids were so expensive. In the past 30 years, however, the technique of meristem culture (a type of tissue culture) has been developed. This results in thousands of identical plants that can be grown on quickly and sold cheaply and is the source of most of the orchids sold in supermarkets and garden centres. The technique must be carried out in sterile conditions and while it is theoretically straightforward, few if any amateur growers attempt it.

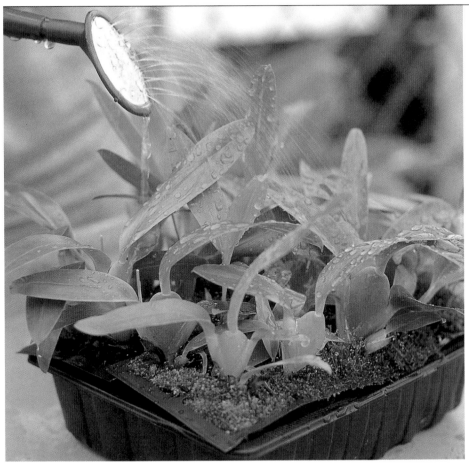

Orchid seedlings growing in a community pot.

Growing from seed

Almost all orchids are insect pollinated and they are often adapted for pollination by only one species of insect. These adaptations vary from something simple like a nectar-filled spur to such bizarre modifications as mimicry, when a flower resembles a female insect and emits a scent resembling the insect's pheromones to attract a male. In the absence of the right insect, we must pollinate a plant ourselves and so long as the orchid has flowers of a reasonable size, this is not too difficult.

The diagrams overleaf show the position of the anther and the stigma in a typical orchid flower. The pollinia, or pollen clumps, which lie under the anther cap, are easily lifted off using a cocktail stick and they should then be placed on the stigma of the same or another flower. The receptive surface of the stigma is sticky and there is rarely a problem in getting the pollinia to adhere to it. It is usually obvious within a few days whether the pollination has worked or not, as the flower starts to go over and the ovary (the part immediately below the flower) shows signs of swelling.

If the aim is to produce seed of a species, it is always best to pollinate the flower of another plant of the same species. Of course this may not be possible and it is always worth trying to self-pollinate a flower if you have only one plant of that species. Some species seem to be self-sterile but more often than not the pollination will succeed, although the resulting seedlings may be fewer in number and less vigorous than

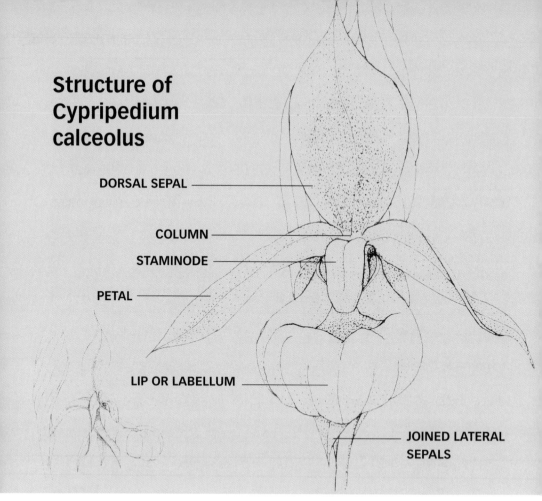

Structure of Cypripedium calceolus

DORSAL SEPAL

COLUMN

STAMINODE

PETAL

LIP OR LABELLUM

JOINED LATERAL SEPALS

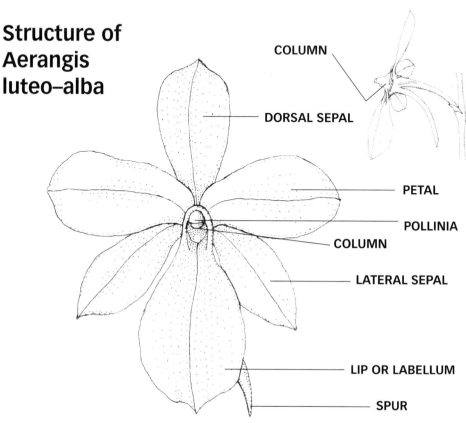

Structure of Aerangis luteo–alba

COLUMN

DORSAL SEPAL

PETAL

POLLINIA

COLUMN

LATERAL SEPAL

LIP OR LABELLUM

SPUR

when two plants are involved. In hybridization, two plants of different species or different hybrids are involved, but the method of pollination is the same. It is important to keep records from which to label and judge the resulting offspring; any developing seed pods should be labelled while still on the plant, giving the names of the plants involved and the date on which the cross was made.

Harvesting the seed

The length of time an orchid seed pod takes to develop varies enormously, from two months to over a year. As a general rule, the larger the seed pod, the longer it takes but there are plenty of exceptions. Usually, when a pod is starting to ripen, it begins to change colour from green to yellowish or pink-ish. When this happens, it is a good idea to remove it from the plant, wrap it loosely in tissue paper and leave it in a warm, dry place until it splits. Then shake out the seed and remove any pieces of pod; these are difficult to sterilize and may act as a focus for infection when the seed comes to be sown.

Seed keeps for a considerable time if it is dry; the easiest way to store it is to keep it in a screw-top jar in a refrigerator with silica gel or some other desiccant in the bottom of the jar.

Orchid seed can also be sown from an unripe seed pod. This is known as 'green podding'. An advantage of this method is that the seed itself does not need to be sterilized, only the outside of the capsule. The capsule should be full size, but not yet ripe; only experi-ence will tell when this has occurred. If capsules, either green or almost ripe, are to be sent through the post it is essential that they are packed in a rigid container so that they do not get crushed. Even ripe seed should be wrapped in something like bubble plastic to give it some protection.

Orchid seed

Orchids produce vast amounts of tiny seeds. The seeds are so small because they do not contain the food reserves found in almost all other seeds. They therefore need a fungus, which may be present in soil or on the bark of a tree, to provide food for growth. Orchid seed can be carried on the wind for great distances and the likelihood of coming across the correct fungus is not high, but so many seeds are produced by one plant that the chances are increased.

Early attempts at seed sowing

In the early days of orchid growing, attempts were made to grow orchids from seed. These were met with little success, until it was found that if the seed was sown around the base of the parent plant, some might germinate and grow on. At the end of the 19th century, Noel Bernard, a French botanist, discovered that orchid seeds were dependent on a fungus for germination and growth. But it was not until the 1920s that Lewis Knudson, an American, discovered that the nutrients provided by the fungus in the wild could be provided artificially by the sower. He experimented with various chemical solutions contain-ing mineral salts and sugars that he added to agar jelly, a substance derived from seaweed. This is the basis of methods used today. As such a nutrient solution is also ideal for the growth of bacteria and fungi, everything, including the seed itself, must be sterilized.

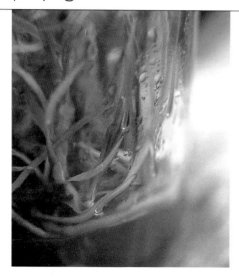

Orchid seedlings in a flask.

Sowing orchid seed

Because of the need for sterile conditions, growing orchids from seed is easier in a laboratory using specially designed equipment, but it can be done successfully using more basic materials such as a pressure cooker and a sterile box or aquarium tank. It is possible to buy nutrient agar so there is no need to make up complicated chemical solutions. The seed is sown into the agar jelly in a glass flask, then the flasks are sealed and kept at a warm, even temperature. Provided all has been kept sterile and the flask is not invaded by fungi or bacteria, you should see signs of the seed developing into what are known as protocorms within a couple of weeks. Protocorms look like lumps of green tissue and they soon develop into tiny plants. As the seedlings grow, they must be replated, that is transferred to a new flask with a fresh and slightly stronger nutrient solution, and grown on again. This also must be done in sterile conditions. There is no space here to go into the methods used in detail; anyone who would like to know more should refer to a book on the subject.

Deflasking

Not many amateur growers attempt to grow orchids from seed themselves, but sooner or later, most find themselves buying orchid seedlings in flasks. For anyone with patience, this is by far the cheapest way to build up a collection. A further advantage is that seedlings in flasks do not need to have CITES permits and plant health certificates, both of which are required when importing mature plants from abroad.

Seedlings grow more quickly in a flask than in a pot and so, in theory, it is a good idea to leave them in the flask as long as possible. However, commercial flasks prepared for sale to the public often have only a thin layer of agar in the bottom and if this has dried up, or if it is filled with roots, then action has to be taken quickly. Likewise, if there are lots of yellow leaves or the seedlings have stopped growing, then it is also time to deflask.

First of all, prepare some pots. Fill some clean plastic pots with a mixture of fine orchid bark and perlite; it is a good idea to put a couple of polystyrene chips in the bottom of the pot to improve the drainage. Stand the bark-filled pots in a sink and pour boiling water over them; this has some sterilizing effect and also washes out most of the fine dust from the bark and perlite. Leave the pots to cool.

Flasks come in many shapes and sizes. Wide-mouthed screw-top jars are frequently used and these are easy to deal with. Prepare a bowl of warm water, open the flask and gently ease the seedlings out into the water. Wash off any agar clinging to the roots; handle the seedlings carefully as leaves and roots break off with alarming ease.

Spread the little plants out on absorbent paper and let them dry off slightly.

Sometimes flasks are bottles of various kinds, and these have to be broken before the seedlings can be extracted. The simplest way is to wrap the bottle in a towel and hit it with a hammer, using just enough force to break the glass but not enough to squash the seedlings inside. Then, wearing gloves, open the towel, pick off the pieces of broken glass and treat the seedlings as before.

We now have seedlings, often with long tangled roots, lying on a piece of absorbent paper. At this point they can be sprayed with a dilute solution of a fungicide/bactericide such as Physan. This is not essential, but it helps to protect the still vulnerable seedlings from infection. The young roots that have grown into the agar never (or hardly ever) turn into adult roots; these grow later from the base of the stem. So the young roots should be trimmed with sterile scissors as otherwise they rot easily, forming a focus for infection, and may also interfere with the growth of the adult roots. Trim the roots down to 2–3 cm (1in) in length, removing any that are very thin or that coil up under the plant.

Community pots

Often the seedlings will be mixed in size and they should be sorted out into more or less matching groups. Plant as many seedlings from each group as possible into one pot because they grow better close together in the early stages. This is known as a community pot.

Now the seedlings must be hardened off before they go into the greenhouse to gradually get them used to the change in climate. A propagator is useful here; they are available in a variety of sizes and most have vents in the lid that can be closed to start with, then opened gradually. Failing that, the community pot can be put into a polythene bag which is sealed at first and then gradually opened to let in air. Results are likely to be much better if seedlings are deflasked in spring or summer, when they grow on quickly.

Seedlings can be left in the community pots for quite a long time. It is usually obvious when they need to be moved on. Either they start to climb out of the pots, with roots waving in the air and finding their way into other pots, or else they stop growing and need the boost that repotting often gives. When they come out of the community pots, they can either be mounted on a bark slab or potted individually. With luck, you will not have to wait too long to see them flower.

While most orchids now in cultivation are artificially bred hybrids, up until the second half of the 19th century only naturally occurring species were grown, which were collected from the wild. The earliest hybrid orchid known to flower was a cross between *Calanthe furcata* and *Calanthe masuca* made by John Dominy, the foreman of the famous orchid nursery Veitch & Sons. He collected seed from this cross in 1854 and a young plant flowered only two years later; it was named *Calanthe* Dominyi. This was not John Dominy's first successful attempt at hybridization; that took place a year earlier and was a cross between two species of *Cattleya*, believed to be *Cattleya guttata* and *Cattleya loddigesii*, but the plants from this cross took six years to flower.

Hybridization

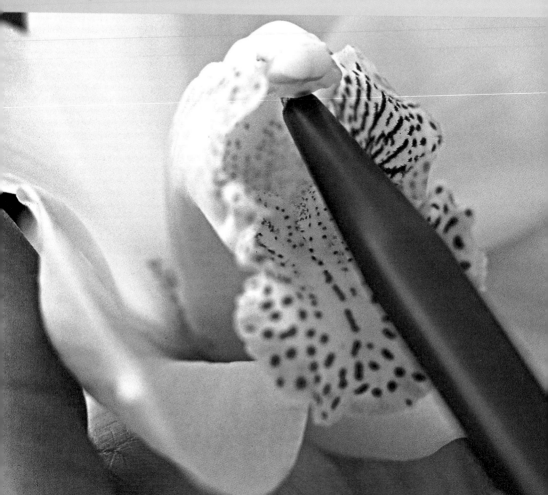

Hybridization

Registration of hybrids

By the end of the 19th century a great many hybrids had been made and had flowered. After 1871, new hybrids were published in the *Gardener's Chronicle*, and from 1893, also in the *Orchid Review* which was established that year.

In 1895 the orchid firm Sander & Sons of St Albans, England, began to register orchid hybrids and in 1906, the first *Sander's List of Orchid Hybrids* was published. Additional volumes appeared at intervals of some years until 1961, when the Royal Horticultural Society became the International Registration Authority. *Sander's List of Orchid Hybrids* is still used today and now the list, containing almost 100,000 names, is available both in print and on compact disc.

Complex hybrids and their names

The first orchid hybrids were between two species of the same genus but it was not long before the first intergeneric cross (between two different genera) was made. This was in 1863, between *Cattleya mossiae* and *Laelia crispa*, to give *Laeliocattleya* Exoniensis. In 1886, *Sophrocattleya* Batemaniana was the result of a cross between *Sophronitis grandiflora* and *Cattleya intermedia*, and in 1892 the first trigeneric hybrid was made: *Sophrolaeliocattleya* Veitchiana, the result of crossing *Sophronitis grandiflora* with *Laeliocattleya* Schilleriana.

So far, the names of intergeneric hybrids had been made by amalgamating the names of the genera involved but as crosses became more complex, involving four or more genera, it became obvious that another way of naming must be found. It was proposed that in

these circumstances, the suffix 'ara' should be added to the name of someone who was involved in either growing or studying orchids.

Among the earliest of such names is *Vuylstekeara* (*Cochlioda* x *Miltonia* x *Odontoglossum*) which was registered in 1911; C. Vuylsteke was a Belgian orchid grower and hybridizer. *Potinara* (*Brassavola* x *Cattleya* x *Laelia* x *Sophronitis*), registered in 1922, is another early name, after M. Potin, a French grower.

These 'manufactured' generic names are written like other generic names in italics and start with a capital letter. The result of a cross between any two species or hybrids is known as a 'grex'. For example, all plants resulting from a cross between *Sophronitis grandiflora* and *Cattleya intermedia* must be called *Sophrocattleya* Batemaniana, regardless of which is the pollen parent and which the seed parent, which varieties were used or when the cross was made. The progeny may look very different and particular forms can be given a cultivar name. Grex names and cultivar names are both written in plain type (not italics) and begin with a capital letter, but the cultivar name is enclosed in single quotation marks; for example, *Vuylstekeara* Cambria 'Plush'. Any awarded plant, whether a species or a hybrid, must be given a cultivar name.

Doing it yourself

Many growers eventually feel the urge to create their own hybrids. Pollination is done in the same way as described in Chapter 5, but if it is to be an intergeneric cross, the genera must be compatible. This usually means that they must be closely related; for example, it is easy to cross *Cattleya* and *Laelia*, but not *Cattleya* with *Cymbidium*. Even so, several attempts may be necessary before the cross is successful.

If you wish to make a serious attempt at hybridization, it is important to have some goal in mind rather than just crossing two plants that happen to be in flower at the same time. The aim might be the production of larger flowers on a more compact plant, for example, or a particular colour of flower. It is necessary to have the space, and patience, to grow many seedlings from the cross on to flowering size – the smallest and slowest might just be the one to have the desired characteristics.

Much is now known about the compatibility of different genera and the inheritance of various characteristics and it is worth reading as much as possible about this before you begin. There is no point wasting years learning from your own mistakes when you could learn very quickly from those of others.

Why grow hybrids?

More people grow hybrid orchids than species. As there are estimated to be over 100,000 registered hybrids with the numbers rising every year, there is plenty of choice. What advantages do hybrids have over species?

The first advantage, not confined to orchids, is what is known as 'hybrid vigour'. Two rather temperamental species can, when crossed, produce a vigorous and easily grown hybrid. As well as growing more quickly, hybrids often flower earlier and more freely and are more tolerant of less than ideal conditions. A grower may want a particular flower colour on a certain size of plant that will grow well in the conditions on offer. It may be difficult to find these characteristics in a species (in fact such a plant may not exist) but it is very likely that there will be a hybrid to fit the bill.

Also, at a more basic level, hybrids are cheaper and more readily available. Like everything else, however, orchids are affected by fashion and this is reflected in the price. The genera which are currently the most popular can be seen by looking at the pages of new registrations which are printed in the *Orchid Review*. Most growers cultivate both hybrids and species although they tend to favour one more than the other. It is perhaps fortunate that there are enough species enthusiasts to keep the raw material for hybrids alive.

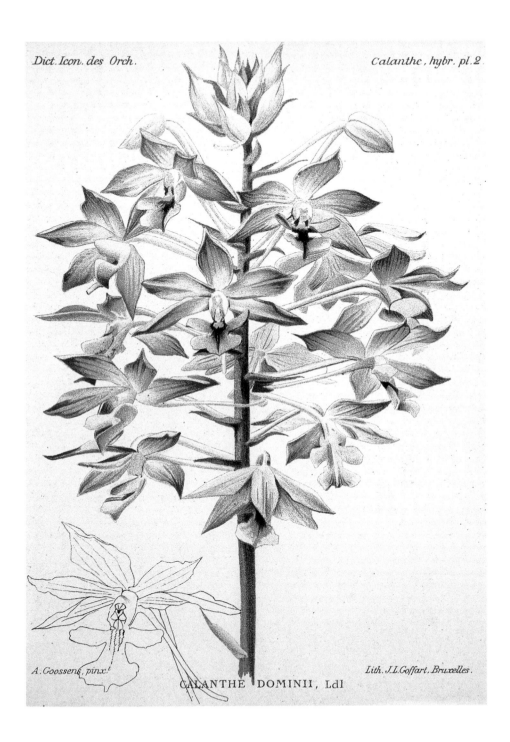

Dict. Icon. des Orch. *Calanthe, hybr. pl. 2.*

A. Goossens, pinx.ᵗ Lith. J.L.Goffart, Bruxelles.

CALANTHE DOMINII, Ldl

Calanthe Dominyi was the first man-made hybrid orchid to flower.

Two of the most frequently grown
and easily available orchids are
suited to cool conditions; these are
cymbidiums and odontoglossums
and their hybrids.

Orchids for the cool greenhouse

minimum night-time temperature **10°C (50°F)**

7

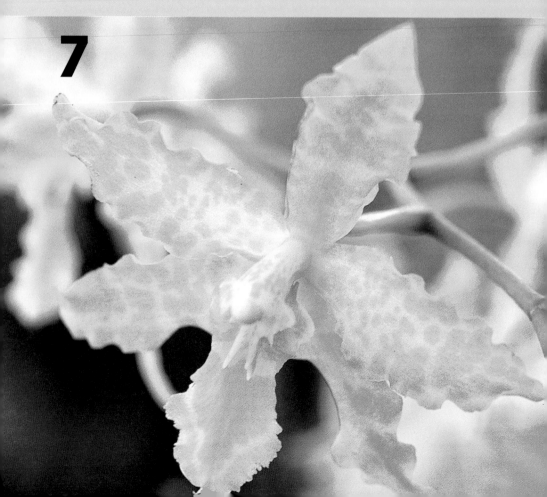

Orchids for the cool greenhouse

Cymbidium

Probably more growers start with a *Cymbidium* than any other type of orchid, as they are widely available and do well as houseplants. There are about 50 species that occur in Asia and Australia but the hybrids are far more widely grown. Cymbidiums need a free-draining compost, usually based on medium bark, and do well in large plastic pots. They are usually bought in flower and although they are easy to grow, it is not always easy to get them to flower the following year. During the summer, they require copious watering and feeding to build up large pseudobulbs. They also need a marked contrast between day and night temperatures – they will not flower without cool nights. The night-time temperature should be about 10°C (50°F) in autumn, winter and spring. It can fall as low as 6°C (43°F) without any harm being done; however, if the night-time temperature rises above about 15°C (59°F), flower buds may drop. In winter, a daytime temperature of 15–18°C (60–65°F) is sufficient; in summer it can rise much higher but the plants will suffer if the temperature is over 30°C (86°F).

Plants benefit from being outside in summer in a bright situation, sheltered from the wind and not exposed to direct sunlight, which can scorch leaves. In winter, they should only be given enough water to prevent the pseudobulbs from shrivelling. Flower stems should be staked soon after they start to develop. Plants should be repotted when the new growths become pressed against the side of the pot. This is best done after flowering or in early spring and they can be divided at the same time. Most need dividing every two to three years.

Dwarf species.

Dwarf *Cymbidium* species have been grown for centuries in China and Japan where their grassy leaves and small, elegant flowers are much appreciated. Special ceramic pots are often used for their cultivation. Some are almost hardy.

C. devonianum

is a species from the Himalayas with pendent flower spikes bearing green flowers heavily marked with purple-red; the lip is pink, spotted with red.

C. erythrostylum,

from Vietnam, has arching flower spikes in spring and summer of up to seven white flowers with a bright yellow lip striped with red.

C. floribundum,

from China and Japan, flowers in spring with erect or arching spikes of many greenish-yellow flowers marked with red or brown. The lip is white with red marks.

C. tigrinum

is a Burmese species with honey-scented green or yellow flowers faintly marked with purple or red and a white lip with purple bars.

Cymbidium 'Bernard Buttercup'

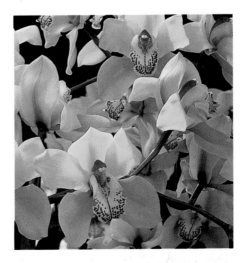

Standard hybrids

These grow into large plants and take up a lot of space, but their spectacular flowers last for up to two months. They are popular as cut flowers and are available in almost every colour except blue. Most flower in late winter and spring. There are hundreds of varieties; there is no space here to mention more than a few.

Caithness 'Cooksbridge', FCC/RHS large, pale green flowers.

Cariga 'Tetra Canary', AM/RHS yellow flower with purple-red marks on the lip.

Coraki 'Red Pauwels' orange-yellow flowers.

Dingwall 'Lewes' white flowers with red-marked lips.

Fort George 'Lewes' , AM/RHS green flowers with purple on the lip; very free flowering.

Howick 'Cooksbridge', AM/RHS large white flowers with a crimson lip.

Many Waters 'Stonehurst', AM/RHS yellow flowers.

Valley Courtier yellow flowers.

Via Abril Roja 'Rose' pink flowers.

Miniature Hybrids

These are mainly derived from the dwarf species described above. They make good houseplants and some have scented flowers. Many have green, yellow or brownish flowers, often with dark marks on the lip, but the range of colours is increasing all the time.

Bulbarrow 'Our Midge' rose red flowers with a darker lip.

Cherry Blossom 'Profusion' only 30cm (12in) tall; pink flowers with darker spots.

Peter Pan 'Greensleeves' scented, green flowers with a crimson lip; autumn flowering.

Stonehaven 'Cooksbridge' cream flowers with yellow and red lip; flowers autumn/winter.

Strathaven usually pink flowers.

Touchstone 'Janis' bronze flowers with a crimson lip.

Hybrids of *C. tigrinum* are mostly green or yellow and appear in spring. They include Wood Nymph, Tiger Cub and Tiger Tail.

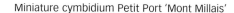

Miniature cymbidium Petit Port 'Mont Millais'

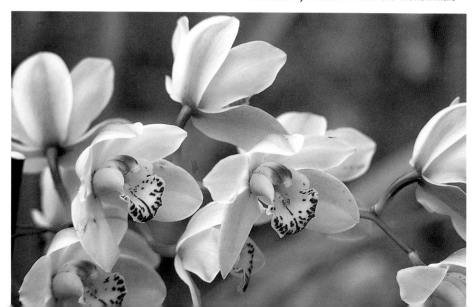

Novelty Hybrids

Some of the best modern hybrids result from a cross between miniature and standard hybrids and are often called novelty or intermediate hybrids – the flowers are as large as those of the standards but the plants are smaller.

Bunny Girl 'Lily White' white flowers, faintly tinged with green.

Calle de Mar 'Green Beauty' green flowers with a crimson lip.

Ivy Fung 'Radiance' mahogany red flowers, edged with cream.

Rincon Fairy 'Pink Perfection' deep pink flowers with red-spotted lips.

Odontoglossum

Most of the 60 species of *Odontoglossum* come from the mountainous areas of Central and South America and so prefer cool temperatures. Grow in a free-draining bark compost with good ventilation and feed and water freely in the growing season. The roots should not remain dry for long periods. They make good houseplants and are slightly unusual in that they tend not to flower at the same time each year but on a nine to ten month cycle, after the new pseudobulb has fully developed.

O. crispum

is a beautiful species from Colombia with many-flowered, arching spikes up to 50cm (20in) long. The flowers have frilly edges, are up to 10cm (4in) in diameter, and are white, often flushed with pink. The lip is marked with yellow and red. There are many awarded clones .

O. harryanum

is another Colombian species with branched flower spikes to 1m (3ft)

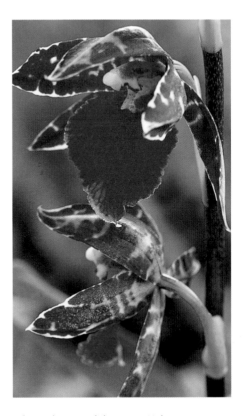

Odontoglossum Violetta von Holme

tall. The flowers grow to 10cm (4in) in diameter; the sepals and petals are yellow, heavily blotched with red-brown, the lip is white with red at its base.

O. odoratum,

from Venezuela, has a flower spike up to 75cm (30in) tall; the scented flowers are about 6cm (21/2in) in diameter, usually yellow spotted with red or brown.

Hybrids

As with *Cymbidium*, the hybrids are more widely grown than the species. *Odontoglossum* belongs to what is known as the Oncidium group of orchids, members of which breed easily with each other, so there are many complex crosses.

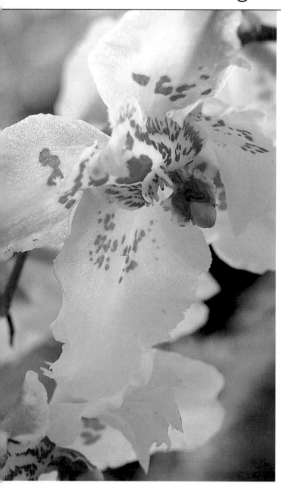

Odontoglossum Marie Kaino

Beallara
(Brassia x Cochlioda x Miltonia x Odontoglossum)
Tahoma Glacier 'Green' a vigorous plant with starry greenish-white flowers with purplish marks on the petals and lip.

Burrageara
(Cochlioda x Miltonia x Odontoglossum x Oncidium)
Living Fire 'Redman' bright red.
Stefan Isler bright red with an orange lip.

Maclellanara
(Brassia x Odontoglossum x Oncidium)
Pagan Lovesong tall spikes of cream or yellow-green flowers with large, brown spots. There are many awarded clones.
Hans Ruedi Isler striking yellow and brown flowers with a red-brown lip.

Odontioda
(Cochlioda x Odontoglossum)
This is the earliest of the crosses between two genera in the Oncidium group, first registered in 1904. Many are predominantly bright red.
Archirondel white flowers with a large maroon blotch on each segment, yellow in the centre.
City of Birmingham yellow flowers with purple and brown marks.
Eric Young large white flowers marked with red.
Heatoniensis star-shaped flowers in pale pink with red spots and a white lip; yellow in the centre. This is one of the earliest crosses.
Honiton Lace 'Burnham', AM/RHS mauve and pink flowers.
Ingmar
orange-red flowers; the sepals and petals are tipped with lilac.
Keighleyensis small, star-shaped, bright red flowers.
Red Rum bright red flowers.
Trixon bright red flowers; the sepals and lip are tinged with lilac, and the lip has a yellow crest.

Odontocidium
(Odontoglossum x Oncidium)
The flower spikes are simple or branched, the flowers varied. Some are rounded, while others have long narrow sepals and petals. The flowers are often boldly marked and the lip can be large or small. Purbeck Gold, Summer Gold, Tiger Butter and Tiger Sun are all yellow with brown markings.

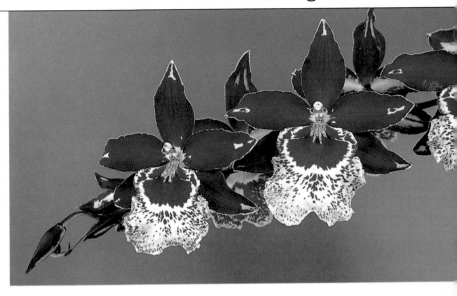

Vuylstekeara Cambria Plush

Odontonia
(Miltonia x Odontoglossum)
An early cross, registered in 1905. Many, but not all, are pastel coloured.

Berlioz 'Lecoufle' large white flowers flushed with mauve-pink, with purple marks radiating from the centre. Several other clones have received awards.

Boussole 'Blanche' pure white flowers with two maroon spots in the centre; free flowering.

Debutante 'Oxbow' brown and yellow flowers with a red and white lip.

Diane bright yellow flowers with brown spots on the sepals and lip; several awarded clones.

Molière very large white flowers sometimes flushed with pink, edged with mauve and with purple marks on the sepals and petals; several awarded clones.

Stewartara
(Ada x Cochlioda x Odontoglossum)
Joyce elegant sprays of bright brown and orange flowers.

Vuylstekeara
(Cochlioda x Miltonia x Odontoglossum)
The flower spikes are simple or branched, the flowers often multi-coloured.

Cambria 'Plush', FCC/RHS the sepals and petals are crimson, the lip white speckled with crimson, with a yellow crest. Said to be the most widely grown orchid in the world.

Jersey basically white flowers, but almost covered with maroon spots; the lip has a yellow crest.

Wilsonara
(Cochlioda x Odontoglossum x Oncidium)
The flower spikes are simple or branched. The flowers are varied but usually rounded in shape and often multicoloured.

Gold Moselle branched sprays of smallish, bright yellow flowers heavily spotted with red-brown.

Kolibri tall, branched sprays of small pink and purple flowers.

Tiger Talk chestnut brown sepals and petals and a golden lip, all tipped with cream.

Widecombe Fair large, branched sprays of small white flowers with purple spots.

Cochlioda

Cochlioda is related to *Oncidium* and *Odontoglossum* and comes from the Andes of Peru, Ecuador and Bolivia. They are small plants with round pseudobulbs, flattened from side to side, with one or two leaves. Grow them in pots with a free-draining compost, with high humidity at cool temperatures. Some species have been used in crosses with *Oncidium* and *Odontoglossum*, where they add red to the colour range. There are six species, but only two are common in cultivation.

C. noezliana
has orange-red flowers 5cm (2in) in diameter, with a yellow callus on the lip and a violet column. It flowers in winter and spring.

C. rosea
has rosy red flowers 3cm (1in) in diameter, with a white callus on the lip, in winter.

Cochlioda rosea

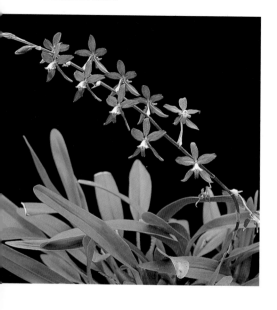

Coelogyne

This large genus of over 100 species from tropical Asia includes several popular, easily grown and free-flowering species. The pseudobulbs are of various shapes and sizes, often large, set close together or well spaced on a woody rhizome. They have one or two leaves and one or many flowers on erect or pendent spikes. Grow in pots or baskets in a fairly coarse bark compost. Those that have pendent flower spikes will need to be hung up while in flower. Water freely while the plants are in active growth but keep almost dry when resting, providing just enough water to keep the pseudobulbs from shrivelling. Most species like good light.

C. cristata
is a popular and rewarding species from the Himalayas with large, round pseudobulbs and pendent spikes of up to ten white flowers with a yellow or orange blotch on the lip, up to 8cm (3in) in diameter. Winter to spring flowers.

C. dayana
is a striking species from Borneo with long, pendent spikes of cream and brown flowers in spring and summer.

C. fimbriata
has short spikes of one to three pale yellow flowers with a fringed lip.

C. massangeana,
with pale yellow and brown flowers, is similar to *C. dayana*.

C. mooreana
is a species from Vietnam with an erect spike of large white flowers with an orange blotch on the lip.

C. nitida
(synonym *C. ochracea*) is a compact, pretty species with erect spikes

of scented white flowers with yellow markings on the lip.

C. ovalis

has beige flowers in autumn; the lip has brownish marks and a fringed margin. This species grows easily and quickly but as the pseudobulbs are set well apart, it tends to climb out of a pot so is better in a basket.

Cypripedium

The temperate slipper orchids are terrestrial plants with deciduous, pleated leaves. The flower structure is similar to that of the tropical slipper orchids, with the lip forming the characteristic pouch. In *Cypripedium*, the edges of the pouch are rolled in. Almost 50 species are known from Europe, Asia and North and South America. Many are fully hardy and can be grown outside in temperate gardens; others are more suitable for alpine house or cool greenhouse culture. Until recently, species have been difficult to obtain as all are strictly protected in the wild, but as more nurseries grow them from seed and growers learn how to accommodate their needs, they are becoming more readily available.

Cypripediums do not have tubers or fleshy roots but a thin, rather woody creeping underground stem that rots if kept too wet and shrivels if kept too dry. Most species like a well-drained soil that is not rich in organic matter. Two suggested compost mixes are:

Mix 1

2 parts medium bark
2 parts fine bark
2 parts leaf mould
2 parts perlite
1 part coarse sand

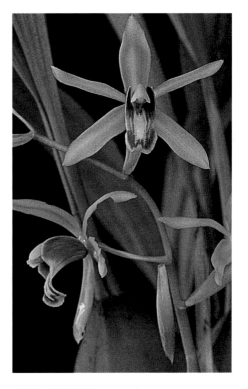

Coelogyne trinerve.

Mix 2

4 parts Seramis
1 part loam (such as John Innes 3)

The following two species are attractive plants for a cool greenhouse.

C. formosanum

has an opposite pair of round, pleated leaves and a white or pale pink flower with darker spots. It flowers in summer.

C. japonicum

grows wild in Japan, Korea and China and is similar to *C. formosanum* but the flowers have pale yellow or yellow-green sepals spotted with purple at the base, and the lip is whitish or yellowish pink, veined and spotted with red. It is rather more temperamental than *C. formosanum*.

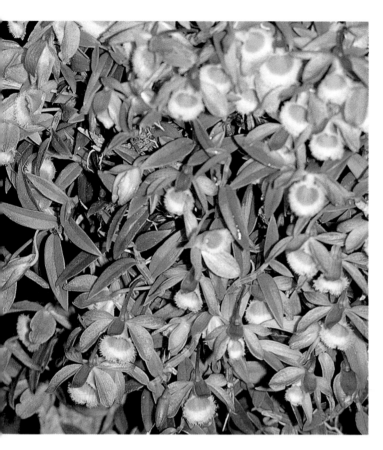

Dendrobium loddigesii

Dendrobium

This is one of the largest of all orchid genera with about 1,000 species widespread in Asia and Australasia. These plants have pseudobulbs of all shapes and sizes and grow in climates ranging from hot, humid tropical lowlands to near alpine conditions on mountains. With such a range, it is difficult to generalize, but while some of the small species grow well mounted on bark, most are grown in baskets or pots (as small as possible) in a fairly coarse, free-draining mix.

Many species, particularly those from India and Australia, like warm, sunny conditions in summer but will not flower unless given cool, dry and bright conditions in winter.

D. aphylla

(synonym *D. pierardii*) is a very pretty species with long, slender, cane-like pseudobulbs, leafy when young but the leaves soon fall. Pale pink flowers, with a primrose yellow trumpet-shaped lip, are borne all along the leafless stems in spring.

D. kingianum

is a widespread Australian species and is one of the easiest of all orchids to grow. Usually 20–30cm (8–12in) tall, it quickly forms dense clumps and has pale to deep pink flowers in winter, although many different colour forms are known.

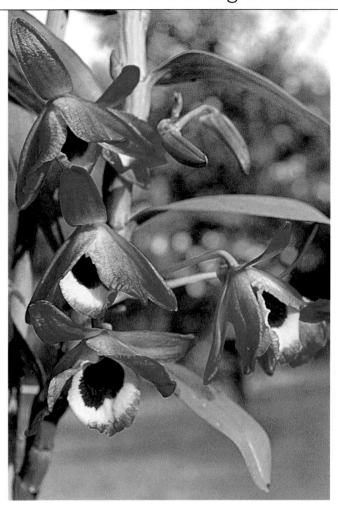

Dendrobium nobile hybrid

If the plant is not properly dried off in winter, it produces keikis on the stems instead of flowers.

D. lindleyi

(synonym *D. aggregatum*) is a small, neat species with rectangular pseudobulbs, short, stiff, oval leaves and pendent clusters of golden yellow flowers.

D. loddigesii

has a creeping habit and is better in a basket or on a raft. When dried off properly in winter, it flowers profusely in spring with lilac flowers with an orange blotch on the lip.

D. nobile

and its hybrids are beautiful plants that are widely grown but they do not flower freely if they are not kept cool and dry in winter. They have clusters of stout canes about 50–75cm (20–30in) tall, with leaves that last for two years. The flowers arise along both leafless and leafy stems. *D. nobile* itself has white or pink flowers about 6cm (2½in) in diameter; the lip has a maroon blotch edged with yellow. The Yamamoto hybrids derived from this species are spectacular plants that come in a wide range of colours.

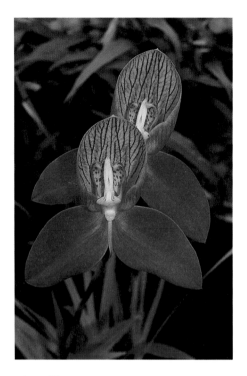

Disa uniflora

Disa

About 130 species of terrestrial orchids from tropical and South Africa with some in Madagascar, but only one species is widely grown. *Disa uniflora* from the Cape Province of South Africa, and its hybrids, are becoming more popular in cultivation as people learn how to grow them.

Disa uniflora

(synonym *D. grandiflora*) grows up to 60cm (24in) tall, with leaves in a rosette at the base and more scattered up the stem, decreasing in size. There are usually from one to three flowers, but occasionally there are as many as ten (in spite of the name), up to 10cm (4in) in diameter, with one of the sepals forming a shallow hood enclosing the petals and the other sepals. The most common

colour is bright red, but yellow and pink forms are known.

Plants often reproduce by stolons and can form large clumps. Unlike most terrestrial orchids, *D. uniflora* never goes completely dormant and should not be dried off. Plants will not tolerate rich soil and need acid conditions (pH 5–6) and very pure water so it is always safer to use rainwater. Try not to get water on to the leaves.

Some growers use completely inert potting composts such as coarse grit; others use a mixture such as sphagnum moss, fibrous peat and chopped bracken. Perhaps the most successful is sphagnum moss alone. As sphagnum tends to deteriorate over time, it is better to repot annually, either in autumn or early spring.

Disa uniflora can withstand temperatures as low as 5°C (40°F), possibly even lower. Good light is important otherwise plants become rather drawn and spindly and the flower colour is less intense.

Plants grown in completely inorganic composts obviously need to be fed, but fertilizer should not be applied at more than one quarter strength, and only when the plants are actively growing in spring and early summer and in autumn when new tubers are being formed. The original tuber that gave rise to the flowering shoot dies after flowering and at least one new tuber is then formed.

Hybrids

The first hybrid, *Disa* Veitchii, (*D. uniflora* x *D. racemosa*) was registered in 1891, but by 1922 only 11 *Disa* hybrids had been registered. In 1981, *Disa* Kirstenbosch Pride (*D. uniflora* x *D. cardinalis*) was registered and this lovely plant seemed to give a boost to further hybridization. By the end of 1995, 135 hybrids had been registered and the number increases each year. Almost all are based on *D. uniflora* and one or more of a mere six or so other species.

They are beautiful plants but most are rather similar in general appearance with tall spikes of orange-red, orange or pink flowers. All should be cultivated in the same way as *D. uniflora*. Good hybrids include:

Betty's Bay

Diores (different cultivars may be pink, red or orange)

Foam

Frieda Duckitt

Helmut Meyer

Kalahari Sands

Kewensis

Kirstenbosch Pride

Langleyensis

Veitchii

Encyclia vitellina

Encyclia

This genus includes about 150 species of orchids from subtropical and tropical America and the West Indies, closely related to *Epidendrum* and at one time included in that genus. Most species have prominent pseudobulbs, usually round or ovoid. The smaller species can be mounted on a bark slab; the larger ones are grown in a shallow pot or a basket in a coarse bark mix. Most species like good light and a dry winter rest.

E. citrina

has grey-green leaves up to 25cm (10in) long and scented, lemon yellow to golden yellow flowers in spring and summer. Although of medium size, this species is better mounted on bark because of its pendulous growth habit.

E. cochleata

is known as the cockleshell orchid because of its shell-shaped lip. Along with some relatives it has recently been transferred to another genus,

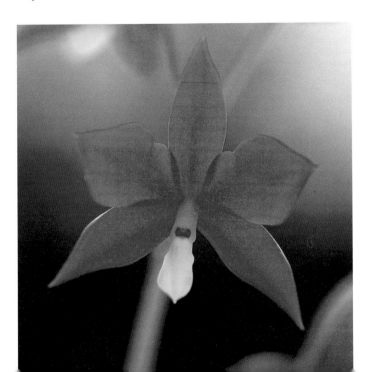

Prosthechea, but it is still usually known as *Encyclia*. The pseudobulbs are large and pear shaped, up to 25cm (10in) long, each with one to three leaves. The flower spike is erect, up to 50cm (20in) tall, with several yellow-green flowers with a deep purple, shell-shaped lip held on top of the flower. The ribbon-like sepals and petals hang down and are about 8cm (3in) long. *E. chacaoensis* is similar to *E. cochleata* with cream or pale green flowers with the lip veined in red.

E. polybulbon

is a dwarf species with small two-leaved pseudobulbs set on a creeping stem. The solitary flowers appear in autumn and winter and are large for such a small plant, with yellow-bronze sepals and petals and a white lip. This species can be mounted or grown in a shallow pan.

E. vitellina

has grey-green leaves and an erect spike of bright orange-red flowers about 3cm (1in) in diameter, in autumn and winter. It is an easy and cheerful plant.

Lemboglossum

There are about 14 species of *Lemboglossum* from Central America and Mexico; they were formerly included in *Odontoglossum*. They have clumps of round or ovoid pseudobulbs. The flowers are showy, of various colours, often barred or spotted. Grow them in shallow pots in a fairly coarse bark mix or mounted on bark.

L. bictoniense

(synonym *Odontoglossum bictoniense*) has an erect, many-flowered spike up to 80cm (32in) tall with scented flowers about 5cm (2in) diameter, usually green-

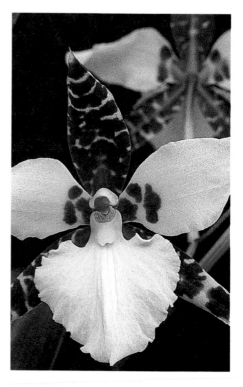

Lemboglossum rossii

ish marked with brown and a white or pink lip. Various colour forms known.

L. cervantesii

(synonym *Odontoglossum cervantesii*) has spikes up to 30cm (12in) tall with two to eight white or pink flowers with broken bands of brown in the lower half, and a white or pink lip with purple stripes at the base. It flowers in winter.

L. rossii

(synonym *Odontoglossum rossii*) is similar to *O. cervantesii* but the sepals and base of the petals are spotted. It flowers in winter.

Lycaste

This genus contains about 45 species found from Mexico through Central America to Peru and Bolivia. The pseudobulbs are large with big, pleated leaves. The long-lasting, erect flowers arise singly at the base of a pseudobulb and have large, spreading sepals. Grow in a coarse bark mix in a shallow pot in light shade. Water and feed freely while growing and provide good ventilation.

L. aromatica
has cinnamon-scented, bright yellow flowers about 8cm (3in) diameter, in winter or spring.

L. lasioglossa
has large orange-brown flowers with a yellow lip, in winter to spring.

L. skinneri
is the National Flower of Guatemala. The flowers are white or pink with a darker lip, up to 15cm (6in) in diameter and appear in winter or early spring. **Jackpot** is a good hybrid with large yellow flowers with darker dots.

Lycaste clinta

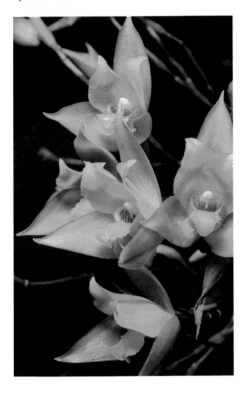

Masdevallia

Masdevallia includes about 350 species of evergreen epiphytic or lithophytic orchids found in Central and South America, often at high altitudes. Their slender stems bear one thick-textured leaf. The sepals are much larger than the petals and lip, and are joined at the base. This results in flowers that are triangular in appearance or more or less tubular, with just the ends of the sepals spreading. The sepals often have long 'tails'. These small plants form dense clumps and often flower off and on throughout the year. They have become very popular with growers as they take up little space and are brightly coloured and free flowering. *Masdevallia* belongs to the Pleurothallid group of orchids.

Most species must have cool conditions and should not be allowed to dry out completely, but are susceptible to rot if overwatered; once this has been mastered, they are easily grown. They are most often grown in a fine bark, usually with perlite and chopped sphagnum mixed in, but can be grown in pure sphagnum moss. Many species can tolerate night-time temperatures as low as 10°C (50°F), but few can withstand temperatures over 26°C (80°F) for more than a short time. They like light shade, high humidity and good air movement. If the humidity can be kept up, they are good windowsill plants.

M. barlaeana
is a medium-sized plant with red, bell-shaped flowers about 4cm (1½in) long.

M. caudata
has scented pink flowers with long yellow tails, mostly in spring.

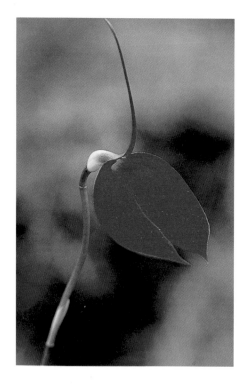

Masdevallia coccinea

M. coccinea

(synonyms *M. harryana* and *M. lindenii*) is a robust and variable species with flowers held well above the leaves. The colour of the long-lasting flowers ranges from white to yellow, red and magenta.

Late spring and summer species
M. coriacea

(synonym *M. uniflora*) is a medium-sized plant with thick leaves and fleshy, cup-shaped flowers, variable in colour but usually white flushed with purple.
M. daviesii

has bright yellow, long-lasting flowers on relatively long stalks.
M. ignea

has yellow, orange or bright red flowers.
M. prodigiosa

has wide apricot or orange flowers with backward-pointing tails, mostly in spring.
M. veitchiana

is a robust and showy plant; flowers are bright orange with bands of purple hairs. Flowers in spring and summer.

Hybrids
Many *Masdevallia* hybrids were made around the end of the 19th century, then few until relatively recently. The hybrids are often more easily grown than the species and flower freely, often off and on throughout the year.
Angel Frost yellow or orange flowers.
Canary yellow or orange flowers.
Copper Angel yellow or orange flowers.
Diana has white flowers with red stripes and yellow tails.
Kimballiana yellow or orange flowers.
Marimba has long-lasting, long-tailed orange to red flowers with darker spots.
Pelican yellow flowers with dark red spots.
Pink Mist in spite of the name, this has creamy flowers tinged with yellow.

Masdevallia **Kimballiana**

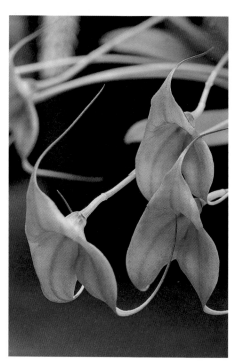

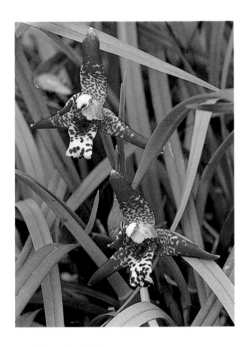

Maxillaria tenuifolia

Maxillaria

There are over 300 species of *Maxillaria* in subtropical and tropical America but relatively few are in cultivation. They are variable in size, with small to large pseudobulbs, usually each with one leaf. Each spike has just one flower in red, brown, yellow or white, which is rarely showy, but interesting. Most are easily grown and do well in an open bark mix in light shade. Keep drier in winter.

M. coccinea
is a dwarf species with a creeping stem and rose pink to scarlet flowers in summer.

M. cucullata
is a variable but free-flowering species; flowers are yellow to brown or almost black, usually striped and spotted with maroon.

M. grandiflora
is one of the bigger species with large, showy, nodding white flowers, which, in the variety *amesiana*, are flushed with pink.

M. picta
has yellow flowers spotted with purple.

M. ubatubana
is similar but a slightly larger plant with bigger flowers.

M. sanderiana
is possibly the showiest species, similar to *M. grandiflora* but the white flowers are 10–15cm (4–6in) in diameter and are marked with red. It is best grown in a basket as the flowers can grow up, down or sideways. Flowers appear in autumn.

M. tenuifolia
is the most widely grown species. It has coconut-scented flowers, usually dark red marked with yellow but sometimes mostly yellow.

Neofinetia

This genus contains one species from Japan and Korea, related to *Angraecum*. Plants can be mounted, but usually do better potted in a fine bark mix. Do not water until the compost has dried out. It will grow in cool or intermediate temperatures, moderate shade and high humidity.

N. falcata

(synonym *Angraecum falcatum*) is a neat plant up to about 20cm (8in) high, often branched at the base and forming clumps. The flowers are white, about 2.5cm (1in) in diameter, with a slender spur, and appear in summer. This species has been widely grown for a long time in Japan, where there are many selected varieties, including ones with pink flowers such as 'Tamahime', and others with variegated leaves. 'Amami Island' has larger flowers than usual.

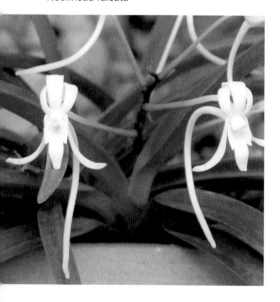

Neofinetia falcata

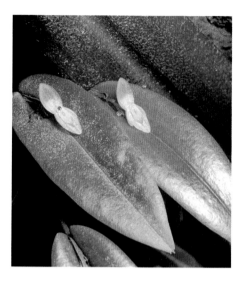

Pleurothallis isthmica

Pleurothallis

A large genus with about 1,000 species found in tropical America. Most are small plants with slender, single-leafed stems and small flowers. Few are showy but they have many enthusiasts. Pot in a fine bark mix or sphagnum; they like high humidity and cool to intermediate temperatures and are very suitable for an orchid case.

P. grobyi

has green, white or yellow-orange flowers, marked with purple or red, in summer.

P. lanceana

has many yellow flowers, tinged with red.

P. schiedii

is a tiny and fascinating species only 2.5–5cm (1–2in) tall. The flowers are light brown and the edges of the sepals are fringed with pendent blobs of white wax.

P. sonderiana

is another tiny plant with lots of long-lasting, small orange flowers.

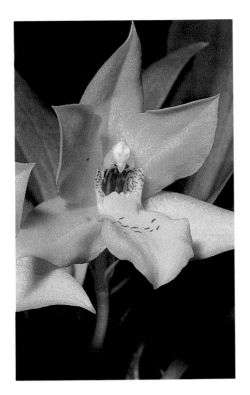

Promenea xanthina

Promenea

There are about 15 species of these dwarf epiphytes found in Brazil. They have small, clustered pseudobulbs, grey-green leaves and relatively large, fleshy flowers. Pot in a free-draining compost.

P. guttata
is less than 8cm (3in) tall; the flowers are bright yellow barred with red, the lip is dark purple at the base, and the tip yellow.

P. stapelioides
has cream to beige flowers, heavily banded with maroon, with a purple lip, in summer.

P. xanthina
(also known as *P. citrina*) has primrose yellow flowers with a bright yellow lip, in summer.

Rossioglossum

This genus contains six species from Mexico and Central America, closely related to *Odontoglossum*. The flowers are large and showy, usually yellow with brown markings. Grow in a standard compost in a shallow pot or basket. Give plenty of water and fertilizer while in growth but keep drier and cooler in winter.

R. grande
(synonym *Odontoglossum grande*) is called the clown orchid. The flower spikes are about 30cm (12in) long, each with about eight flowers. The flowers are 15cm (6in) in diameter with yellow sepals, barred and dotted with chestnut brown. The petals are yellow with a brown base and the lip is cream or pale yellow, banded with red and brown. The yellow and red callus is supposed to resemble a clown. Flowers appear in autumn and winter.

Rossioglossum grande

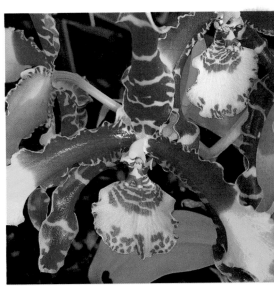

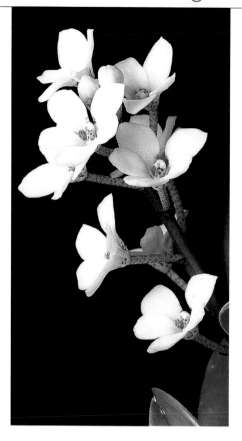

Sarcochilus hartmannii

Sarcochilus

This genus comprises about 15 species of dwarf orchids from Australia and South East Asia. They are compact plants that can be mounted on bark or potted in a fairly coarse mix and like light shade and high humidity with good air movement.

S. hartmannii
has stems that branch at the base to form clumps. The waxy white flowers are spotted with maroon in the centre and are up to 3cm (1in) in diameter. They are good plants for a windowsill or orchid case.

Sophronitis

About seven dwarf species from high altitudes in Bolivia, Paraguay and eastern Brazil. The flowers are showy, large for the size of plant, usually red but some-times bright pink or orange. They like shady, humid conditions and good venti-lation and can be grown in small pots in fine bark compost or mounted on a slab. They are slow to establish and should be divided as little as possible; a well-established plant is a spectacular mass of colour when in flower.

Species of *Sophronitis* have been much used in hybridization with relatives such as *Cattleya* and *Laelia* for the small size and bright colours they bring to a cross.

Sophrocattleya Jewel Box 'Darkwaters'

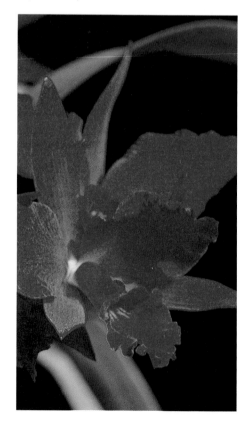

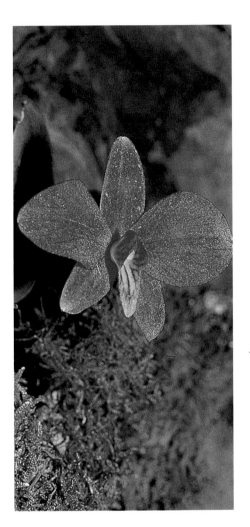

Sophronitis coccinea (synonym *S. grandiflora*)

S. cernua
has orange-red flowers about 3cm (1in) in diameter.

S. coccinea
(synonym *S. grandiflora*) is a free-flowering plant with fleshy flowers 8cm (3in) in diameter, usually bright scarlet with yellow at the base of the lip, but other colour forms exist. The variety *aurantiaca* is orange, *purpurea* is purple and *rossiteriana* is yellow. Flowers are borne in winter.

Stenoglottis

Five or six species of *Stenoglottis* are known from tropical East Africa and South Africa. They are quite small plants with cylindrical, tuberous roots; the leaves form a rosette with the flower spike arising in the centre. All the species look rather similar and all are easily grown, attractive plants that do well in a cool greenhouse or on a windowsill.In the wild, they often grow in a thin layer of moss or soil on top of a rock but do well in a free-draining terrestrial compost or a fine bark mix. After flowering, or sometimes even while the plant is still in flower, the leaves start to die back. Pick off the dead leaves and keep the plant dry until signs of new growth appear, usually after two or three months.Stenoglottis plants can be easily propagated by division. Each tuberous root has a growing point at one end, but they look better when allowed to form a good clump.

S. fimbriata
has attractive, wavy-edged leaves, heavily spotted with purple. The late summer flowers are pink with a three-lobed, purple-spotted fringed lip.

S. longifolia
is the tallest species, with a flower spike reaching up to 50cm (20in), and is the most common in cultivation. The leaves are plain green often with wavy edges; the autumn flowers are pink with a purple-spotted, five-lobed lip.

S. woodii
is a small plant; the flower spike grows up to 20cm (8in) tall. The leaves are plain green, the flowers are usually white but there is a pink form. It flowers in summer, earlier than the other species.

The most popular orchids that are suitable for an intermediate greenhouse are cattleyas and laelias and their hybrids, *Miltoniopsis* hybrids (pansy orchids), *Phalaenopsis* (moth orchids) and paphiopedilums (slipper orchids), but many other orchids will also grow happily in these conditions.

Orchids for the intermediate greenhouse
minimum night-time temperature 15°C(60°F)

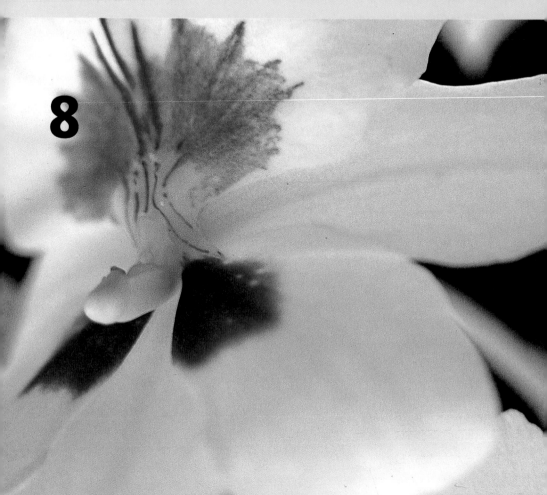

8

Orchids for the intermediate greenhouse

Aerangis

African orchids are increasing in popularity and species of *Aerangis* are among the most desirable. There are about 50 species in Africa and Madagascar; most are small or medium in size. The leaves are usually thick-textured, in most species wider near the apex than the base.

They have arching or pendent spikes of elegantly shaped, spurred white flowers sometimes tinged with salmon pink or rusty red, almost all strongly and sweetly scented at night. With a few exceptions, they like shady, humid conditions with good air movement. They do well mounted on bark provided the humidity is high enough, but they will grow in pots in a free-draining compost. Almost all thrive in intermediate conditions, and any species that can be obtained is worth growing.

A. articulata,
from Madagascar, has greyish-green leaves often edged with reddish-purple and long sprays of pure white flowers.

A. brachycarpa
is one of the larger species from tropical Africa. It has dark green, luxuriant leaves and long sprays of white flowers.
A. confusa, from Kenya, is similar but has slightly smaller, more strongly pink-tinged flowers. It is very reliable and sometimes flowers twice a year.

A. citrata
is a small species from Madagascar with long sprays of creamy white, occasionally creamy yellow flowers, very freely borne.

A. distincta,
from Malawi, was only described in

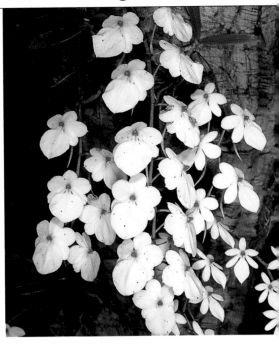

Aerangis luteoalba var. *rhodosticta*

1987 but is already well established in cultivation. The leaves are deeply bilobed at the tip, resembling a fish tail. The flowers are large with pink-tipped sepals and long spurs. There are two forms, one flowering in spring, the other in late summer.

A. fastuosa
is a small species from Madagascar, with dark green leaves, that produces a mass of large, pure white flowers on shorter spikes than most.

A. kotschyana
is a tropical African species with broad, dark green leaves and long sprays of white flowers with a salmon pink spur up to 25cm (10in) long with a corkscrew twist in the middle. Intermediate to warm conditions required with moderate shade; keep drier in winter. This species does better when mounted; if it is potted, the compost should be coarse and free-draining.

A. luteoalba var. rhodosticta
is a small but very distinctive species from East Africa that flowers from an early age. The leaves are narrow and

dark green; flowers are creamy white with a red column.

A. mystacidii

is another of the smaller species but is free flowering and reliable. It is a neat plant with dark green leaves and white, pink-tinged flowers with a spur up to 8cm (3in) long.

A. verdickii

is a distinctive species from East Africa with fleshy, grey-green leaves, often with undulating, purple edges. The strongly scented flowers are white with spurs up to 20cm (8in) long. The thick roots and succulent leaves show that this species is adapted to a harsh dry season and it should be kept almost dry when not in active growth. It likes only light shade and is better mounted; again, if potted it should be in a very coarse mix.

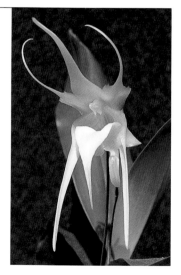

Aeranthes caudata

Aeranthes

There are 30–40 species of *Aeranthes* in Madagascar and the other Indian Ocean islands, with two species in Zimbabwe. They appeal to people who like strange flowers; they are not conventionally showy but always attract attention when in flower. They have short stems and leaves forming a fan. The flowers are green, yellow-green or greenish-white and are usually borne dangling on long, wiry, pendent spikes. Most have fine roots and grow better in a pot in a fairly fine compost. Hang up when the plant is in flower. They prefer humid, shady conditions.

A. grandiflora

has bright green leaves and yellow-green or greenish-white flowers. *A. arachnites* is similar but slightly smaller.

A. henricii

looks very different from all other *Aeranthes* species. The leaves are dark green, the roots thick and often flattened. The flowers are green and white, almost 20cm (8in) in diameter, with a slender spur 15cm (6in) long. It is a striking plant but can be reluctant to flower.

Aerangis mystacidii

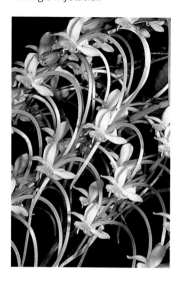

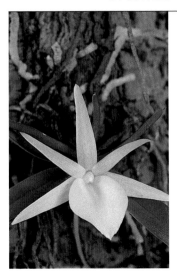

Angraecum didieri

Angraecum

There are about 200 species of *Angraecum* in Africa and Madagascar, which range in size from very small to very large. They have white, green or yellow-green flowers with a long or short spur. Species with white, long-spurred flowers are pollinated by night-flying moths and are strongly scented in the evening and at night. Most species grow well in pots in a medium or coarse bark mix, depending on size.

A. calceolus
is a compact, medium-sized plant with branched spikes of yellow-green flowers. It is not showy but is easily grown and rarely out of flower.

A. compactum
is a neat plant with dark green leaves and large, pure white flowers. It likes a humid, shady situation.

A. didieri
is one of the best species for anyone who is short of space. The plants are small with narrow, dark green leaves and warty roots. The flowers are large for the size of plant, and are pure white with long spurs. It likes moderate shade and grows well mounted provided the

humidity is high; otherwise pot in medium bark. *A. rutenbergianum* is similar but has slightly smaller flowers.

A. germinyanum
is a variable species with long, slender stems and white flowers with a shell-shaped lip held uppermost; the sepals and petals are long and spidery; the spur is long and slender. It grows well potted or mounted in shady, humid conditions.

A. leonis
has a short stem with a fan of fleshy, flattened leaves. The flowers are large and white with a funnel-shaped lip at the base and a long spur.

A. magdalenae
is one of the finest species. It is a medium-sized plant with dark green leaves forming a fan and large, pure white flowers with a strong, spicy scent in the evening. In the wild it grows on rocks in only light shade, and so it prefers good light. Pot in a coarse mix and keep drier in winter.

A. sesquipedale,
the comet orchid, is one of the best known species. The medium to large plants have large, waxy, creamy-white flowers with a spur up to 30cm (12in) long, in winter. It thrives in warmer parts of an intermediate house, in good light.

Angraecum sesquipedale

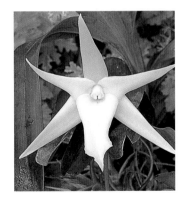

Anguloa

About ten species of *Anguloa* occur in the South American Andes. They are large plants, related to *Lycaste*, with big pseudobulbs and pleated leaves which last for only one season. The flowers are cup-shaped, usually yellow, and sometimes marked with red-brown. Flowers are produced singly at the base of a pseudobulb. Plants require ample feeding and water while in growth but should be kept almost dry while dormant. They should be grown in the cooler parts of an intermediate house.

Anguloa clowesii

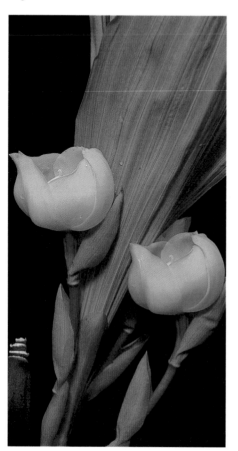

A. clowesii
has scented lemon or golden yellow flowers.
A. uniflora
has creamy white flowers flushed with pink and with red spots near the base.

Angulocaste
(Anguloa x Lycaste)

These are large plants with very big, pleated leaves. They have one or two tulip-shaped flowers on long stems arising from the base of plant. They require shady, intermediate conditions; keep them dry in winter.

Andromeda large pink flowers spotted with red.
Apollo 'Goldcourt' greenish-yellow flowers with red spots.
Aurora red and orange flowers.
Gemini mahogany-red sepals and creamy yellow petals dotted with red.
Wyld Charm deep pink flowers.
Wyld Delight scented yellow flowers with red dots.

Angulocaste Apollo

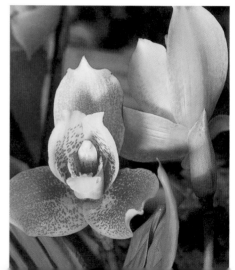

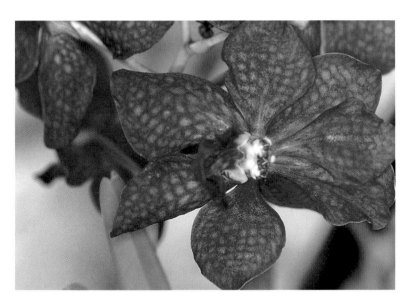

Ascocenda Princess Mikasa

Ascocenda
(Ascocentrum x Vanda)

These hybrids have become very popular as they require less light to flower, tolerate lower temperatures and are smaller plants than vandas, but have larger flowers than ascocentrums. The flowers are brightly coloured and long lasting. Here are a few of the named hybrids available:

Bangkok freely produced orange-peach flowers with an orange-red lip.

Dong Tarn bright red flowers with maroon spots.

Madame Nok yellow flowers with dark red spots; the mid lobe of the lip is red.

Meda Arnold deep pink or red flowers.

Pak-Chong lime green flowers with a white column.

Princess Mikasa 'Blue Velvet' deep violet blue flowers.

Suk Samran Beauty 'Surat Pink', AM/RHT large pink flowers.

Sunkist yellow flowers.

Tan Chai Beng 'Violet Delight' violet flowers.

Tubtim Velvet white flowers, tipped with pink.

Udomchai orange flowers.

Yip Sum Wah smallish but vivid orange flowers.

Brassavola

This genus includes about 15 species of orchid in tropical America, related to *Cattleya*. They have small pseudobulbs with one fleshy leaf at the apex and medium-sized or large green and white flowers, scented in the evening. They prefer good light and can be mounted or grown in pots or baskets. They like cool to intermediate night-time temperatures, but do not mind high daytime temperatures. Species of *Brassavola* have been used a lot in hybridization with *Cattleya* and other relatives.

B. cucullata
has pendent leaves up to 25cm (10in) long and large, greenish-white flowers in autumn with long, drooping sepals and

petals. The lip has a long, slender tip.

B. digbyana

See *Rhyncholaelia digbyana*.

B. nodosa

(synonym *B. venosa*) This attractive species has large, greenish-white or cream flowers with a white lip, strongly scented in the evening. Flowers are borne in winter.

B. tuberculata

(synonyms *B. fragrans* and *B. perrinii*) This plant has long leaves that are almost cylindrical, but grooved on top. The summer flowers are creamy yellow or lime-green, sometimes with red spots, and a white lip, sometimes with green or yellow in the throat.

Brassia

This genus includes about 25 species of epiphytic orchid from tropical America. The ovoid pseudobulbs each have one or two leaves and the plants bear large, spidery, showy flowers with long, narrow sepals and petals. Grow them in coarse bark in a pot or basket; feed and water freely in summer but keep almost dry in winter.

B. caudata

has arched flower spikes up to 80cm (32in) long with the flowers in two rows. The summer flowers are yellow or orange, usually marked with red-brown; the lip is yellow or green. The lateral sepals have long, slender tails up to 18cm (7in) long.

Brassia verrucosa

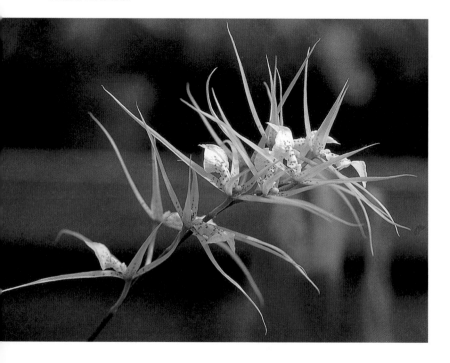

B. maculata

has yellow-green flowers with purple marks in early summer.

B. verrucosa

has pale yellow to lime green flowers with brown spots. The white lip has red spots at the base and prominent green warts; the sepals are up to 12cm (5in) long. Flowers appear in spring and early summer.

B. Rex
(B. verrucosa x gireoudiana)

has spidery flowers larger than those of either parent, in pale green with brown spots and green warts. Many cultivars have received awards, including 'Barbara', AM/AOS and 'Tacoma', AM/AOS.

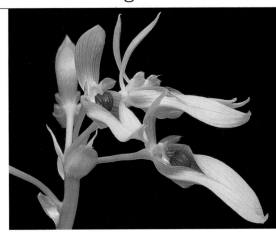

Bulbophyllum graveolens

Bulbophyllum

With over 1,000 species found throughout the tropics, this is one of the largest orchid genera. Plants have a creeping, woody stem with large or small pseudobulbs set either close together or well spaced out, each with one or two thick-textured leaves. The flowers vary from showy to small and dull-coloured, but many are bizarrely shaped and often attract attention. Species in the section *Cirrhopetalum* (originally a genus in its own right and still considered as such by some authorities) have large flowers coming off at almost the same height at the top of the flowering stem.

Species where the pseudobulbs form clumps do well potted in a fine but well-drained bark mix, but when the pseudobulbs are set far apart, plants keep climbing out of a pot and are better in a basket or on a slab of bark. In the wild they occur at a wide range of altitudes but in cultivation most will grow in intermediate temperatures. Most like good light and should be kept fairly dry when not actively growing; they should be watered with care while new growth is developing as that tends to rot with too much moisture.

B. barbigerum

is a small West African species with round, flat, pale green, single-leafed pseudobulbs and deep maroon-purple flowers in summer. The lip is fringed with long hairs clubbed at the tips. It does better mounted.

B. lobbii

is a striking species from South East Asia. The large summer flowers are usually yellow, streaked and spotted with red-brown.

B. longiflorum

(synonym *Cirrhopetalum umbellatum*) is a widespread species found from Africa through Asia to Australia. The flowers are about 3cm (1in) long, usually mottled light and dark purple, but sometimes they are bronze or clear yellow.

B. macranthum

is a large-flowered species from Burma with yellowish or speckled purple flowers about 5cm (2in) in diameter in early summer.

B. medusae

(synonym *Cirrhopetalum medusae*) is
a species from South East Asia with
round heads of spidery cream flowers
with a strange, tangled appearance,
in winter.

B. rothschildianum

(synonym *Cirrhopetalum rothschildianum*), from India, has striking
but unpleasant-smelling, maroon
flowers mottled with yellow, in winter.

B. sandersonii

is an African species in which part of
the flower spike is swollen but flattened,
and often purple. The deep purple,
occasionally yellow, flowers are
arranged along either side. It is a
strange-looking plant that always
causes comment when it is in flower.
B. scaberulum and *B. purpureorhachis*
are similar in general appearance.

Hybrids

Several hybrids exist, most involving
species in section *Cirrhopetalum*, but
only one seems to be readily available.

Bulbophyllum Elizabeth Ann
(B. longissimum x
B. rothschildianum)

has pendent sprays of pink-mauve
flowers. The cultivar 'Bucklebury' is out-
standing and has received an AM from
both the RHS and the AOS.

Calanthe

This genus includes about 150 species
of medium to large terrestrial orchids
found in tropical and subtropical Africa,
Asia and Australia, with most species in
Asia. The pseudobulbs are small to large;
the evergreen or deciduous leaves are
pleated. Plants need a free-draining terrestrial compost and a shady position;
they do better if repotted every year in
spring. The deciduous species grow at
intermediate temperatures but the
evergreen species are more suited to
an alpine house. They seem to have
been more widely grown in the past
than they are now.

Deciduous species

These should be kept dry in a cool, bright
place after the leaves are shed, or they
will not flower. The flowers appear in
late winter, before the leaves.

C. rosea

has pink flowers with a darker lip.

C. vestita

is widespread in South East Asia. The
flowers are creamy white with a yellow
blotch on the lip but there are many

Calanthe St. Brelade

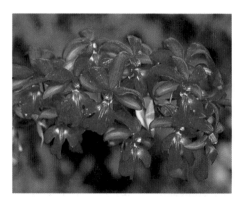

colour forms, including the variety *rubro-maculata* with a red-purple blotch on the lip and *williamsii*, which is pale pink with a crimson lip.

Hybrids

Many attractive hybrids are available and most are rather large plants.
Diana Broughton deep rose pink.
Sedenii white.
Veitchii pale pink.
William Murray white with a red-purple blotch on the lip.

Cattleya

Cattleyas are the stereotypical orchids and used to be very popular as corsages. There are about 50 species in tropical Central and South America. Most have large pseudobulbs with one or two leaves each, set on a stout, creeping stem. The flowers are large and showy, with spreading sepals and petals and a lip that is often trumpet-shaped with frilly edges. They are usually grown in wide, shallow pots or baskets in a coarse bark mix and like good light. They need plenty of water and fertilizer while in growth and a drier, cooler rest in winter. The leaves enclose a sheath from which flowers appear. Cattleyas are divided into unifoliate (single-leafed) and bifoliate (two-leaved) species.

Unifoliate species
C. labiata
was the first of the large-flowered species to be brought into cultivation. The flowers are as large as 15cm (6in) in diameter, typically pale to deep pink with a magenta lip with a yellow blotch at the base, but there are many named and awarded varieties. All flower in autumn.

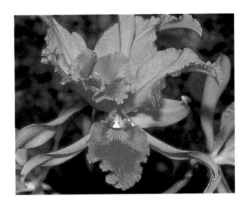

Cattleya labiata

C. eldorado, *C. gaskelliana*, *C. perce-valiana*, *C. warneri* and *C. warscewiczii* are all rather similar and are often confused with *C. labiata*.
C. maxima
is a species from Ecuador, Colombia and Peru with large, lilac-pink flowers. The lip has purple veins and a yellow mark in the throat. It flowers in winter.

Bifoliate species
These species need a slightly longer winter rest. They tend to be smaller plants than the unifoliate species.
C. amethystoglossa
has up to 20 flowers on the spike, each about 10cm (4in) in diameter. The sepals and petals are white or pale pink with purple spots; the lip is magenta. Flowers appear in spring.
C. aurantiaca
is a free-flowering Central American species with relatively small, bright orange flowers in summer.
C. bicolor
is an elegant species from Brazil with flowers up to 9cm (3½in) in diameter. The sepals and petals are greenish-bronze, the lip is magenta-purple. Late summer to autumn flowers.

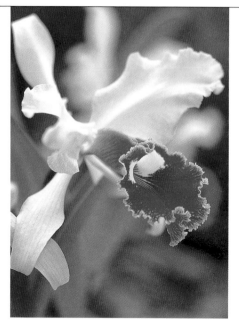

Cattleya trianaei

C. intermedia

has large, strongly scented flowers with lilac or white sepals and petals and a purple, lilac or white lip in summer.

C. skinneri

is the National Flower of Costa Rica. It has rose pink or purple flowers in early summer and is a good windowsill plant.

Hybrids

These are so numerous it is possible to mention only a very few.

Angel Bells white flowers.

Bob Betts 'White Wings' large, well-shaped white flowers in spring.

Bow Bells white flowers with a yellow blotch in the throat in autumn.

Chocolate Drop many smallish, orange-red flowers.

Dale Edward salmon pink flowers.

Guatemalensis smallish, salmon pink flowers in spring. A natural hybrid.

Lamartine white flowers with a gold lip, edged with pink.

Portia 'Coerulea' lavender blue flowers in autumn.

Intergeneric hybrids

All *Cattleya* species are beautiful but many make large, sprawling plants. They have been extensively crossed with related genera, such as *Brassavola*, *Epidendrum*, *Laelia* and *Sophronitis*, and many of the hybrids, particularly more recent ones, produce large flowers on compact plants, sometimes called mini-cattleyas or mini-cats. Hybrids involving *Sophronitis* tend to be compact plants with relatively large, brightly coloured flowers.

Brassocattleya
(Brassavola x Cattleya)

Fuchs Star starry white flowers with a broad lip veined with mauve.

Pluto large, strongly scented pale green flowers with a fringed lip.

Touraine white flowers; the lip is large and edged with mauve.

Brassolaeliocattleya
(Brassavola x Cattleya x Laelia)

Fortune yellow with a red lip.

Good as Gold bright yellow.

Jungle Treasure miniature plant; yellow flowers with a red lip.

Cattleya aurantiaca

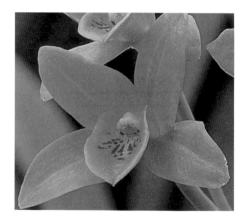

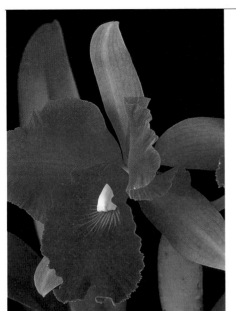

Potinaria Sunrise

Pumpkin Festival bright red flowers.
Yellow Imp 'Golden Grail', AM/AOS –
bright yellow.

Laeliocattleya
(*Cattleya* x *Laelia*)
These plants come in a range of colours.
Angel Heart 'Hihimauu' Pink and
white scented flowers, marked with
darker pink.
Barbara Belle 'Apricot' apricot
yellow flowers.
Beaumesnil 'Parme' bright magenta
flowers with a yellow lip and purple
stripes.
Daniris large yellow flowers with a
purple and gold lip.
El Corrito yellow flowers.
Georges Issaly large, mauve flowers.
Irene Finney mauve flowers with a
darker lip.
Schilleriana
a natural hybrid between *Laelia purpu-
rata* and *Cattleya intermedia*; usually
white with a purple lip but there are
other colour forms.
Stradivarius 'Eclipse' salmon pink
with a yellow lip.

Tropical Pointer 'Cheetah' orange
with brown spots.

Potinara
(*Brassavola* x *Cattleya* x *Laelia* x
Sophronitis)
Haw Yuan Gold 'D-J' rich golden
yellow flowers.
Sunrise light magenta flowers with a
darker lip, orange at the base.

Sophrocattleya
(*Cattleya* x *Sophronitis*)
Angel Face miniature; bright pink
flowers with a pink-fringed yellow lip.
Crystelle Smith 'Nathan's Reward',
HCC/AOS bright pink flowers with a
yellow lip.

Sophrolaeliocattleya
(*Cattleya* x *Laelia* x *Sophronitis*)
Coastal Sunrise has several cultivars
including 'Lemon Chiffon' (yellow), 'Pink
Surprise' (pinkish-purple) and 'Tropico',
HCC/AOS (orange, tinged with purple).
Epsom miniature; pink flowers with a
darker lip.
Ginny Champion 'Prince' miniature;
orange-red flowers, yellow in the centre
with a red lip.
Hazel Boyd 'Royal Scarlet' semi-
miniature plant; bright red and orange,
free-flowering.
Jewel Box 'Sheherezade' carmine red
flowers with a darker lip.
Jungle Bean bright yellow flowers with
a red lip.
Roblar 'Orange Gem' small, bright
orange flowers.
Sutter Creek 'Gold Country',
HCC/AOS – miniature plant with bright
yellow flowers with red-fringed lips.
Tiny Titan miniature; flowers may be
yellow, orange or red, with a red lip.

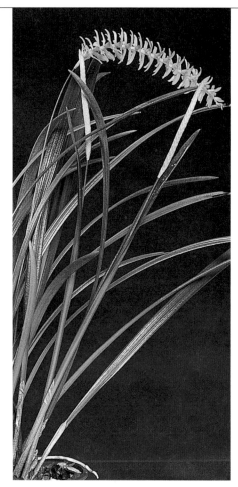

Dendrochilum javierense

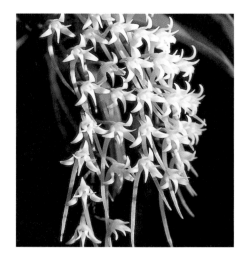

Cyrtorchis praetermissa

Cyrtorchis

Cyrtorchis contains about 15 species of monopodial, epiphytic orchids from tropical Africa and South Africa with waxy, white, scented flowers, with long spurs. Most have thick roots and glossy, bright green leaves. Grow mounted or in pots or baskets in a coarse bark mix, in moderate shade at intermediate temperatures.

C. arcuata
is a widespread species with a woody stem and creamy white flowers 5cm (2in) in diameter. Subspecies *whytei* has broader leaves, larger flowers and a longer spur, up to 10cm (4in) long.

C. chailluana
is the largest species with spidery flowers up to 7.5cm (3in) in diameter and a slender spur to 15cm (6in) long.

C. praetermissa
is a small species with dark green, folded leaves; the spikes have two rows of creamy white flowers with a lily-of-the-valley scent.

Dendrochilum

This genus contains about 120 species of epiphytic orchid from South East Asia, sometimes known as necklace orchids or golden chain orchids. The pseudo-bulbs often form clumps and are of various shapes with one or two leaves each. The flower spikes are graceful, erect at first then arching, with many small flowers. Many species are worth growing but only a few appear in cultivation. They do well in shallow pots with a medium, free-draining compost and are better with a short winter rest. Those with very long spikes need to be suspended when in flower.

D. cobbianum
has conical, single-leafed pseudobulbs and long spikes of white flowers with a yellow lip in autumn.

D. filiforme
has small, clustered pseudobulbs each with two narrow leaves. The slender spike has many scented, yellow flowers in summer.

D. glumaceum
has larger flowers than most. They are white, scented, have large, cream bracts and appear in spring. *D. latifolium* is similar but more vigorous and with smaller bracts.

Epidendrum

There are about 500 species of *Epidendrum* in tropical America. The plants are very variable in size and manner of growth. Some are small, creeping plants while others have tall, reed-like stems. Most species with distinct pseudobulbs are now included in *Encyclia*. Most are epiphytic but a few are terrestrial and some grow on rocks. Apart from small species that are better mounted, they grow well in pots in a bark mix and in an intermediate greenhouse.

E. cinnabarinum
has cane-like stems up to 1m (3ft) tall with many bright orange-red flowers up to 6cm (2½in) across.

E. ibaguense
(synonym *E. radicans*) is a tall plant with cane-like, leafy stems 1–1.5m (3–5ft) high and red flowers with a fringed lip. *E. O'brienianum* is an early hybrid of this species which is widely grown; it is similar with rose red flowers. These plants are easily grown in cool or intermediate

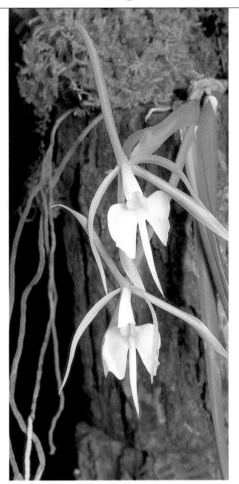
Epidendrum parkinsonianum

conditions, in good light, and flower almost all year round. They are often grown in tropical gardens.

E. parkinsonianum
has narrow, fleshy, pendent leaves 30–50cm (12–20in) long. The flowers are large, scented and long lasting, with yellow-green sepals and petals and a pure white lip. Because of the pendent leaves, it needs to be mounted on bark or in a suspended pot in a coarse bark mix. It prefers fairly good light.

E. porpax
is a small, creeping plant with fleshy yellow-green flowers with a purple lip.

E. pseudepidendrum
is a tall species with lime green sepals and petals and a glossy, bright orange lip. It flowers in winter.

Eulophia

Over 200 species of terrestrial orchids found throughout the tropics and subtropics, with most in tropical and South Africa. Some have chains of underground corms while others have pseudobulbs partly above ground, usually forming clumps; the latter tend to be easier to grow. There are many beautiful species, but unfortunately only a few are available in cultivation. All species have fleshy roots that rot easily, so they need a free-draining compost which should be allowed to dry out before watering again. Plants should be kept dry in winter until signs of new growth are seen in

spring, when careful watering can start again. As with all terrestrial orchids, it is vitally important to follow the plant's own rhythm. All seem to do well in intermediate conditions in fairly good light.

E. euglossa

has conical, glossy green pseudobulbs up to 20cm (8in) long. The flower spike grows up to 1m (3ft) tall, and bears many green flowers with a white lip veined with pink. Flowers appear in summer. This is a forest plant and appreciates slightly more shade than other species.

E. guineensis

(synonym *E. quartiniana*) has small pseudobulbs and broad, pleated leaves. The flower spike is 30–50cm (12–20in) tall, the flowers are about 5cm (2in) in diameter with narrow, erect, green or purple-brown sepals and petals and a large pink lip with a purple blotch at the base. Flowers are borne in summer.

E. streptopetala

(synonym *E. paiveana*) has ovoid, ribbed pseudobulbs up to 10cm (4in) tall and pleated leaves up to 60cm (24in) long. The spike is 1–1.5m (3–5ft) tall, with many yellow and purple-brown flowers in summer.

Eulophia guineensis

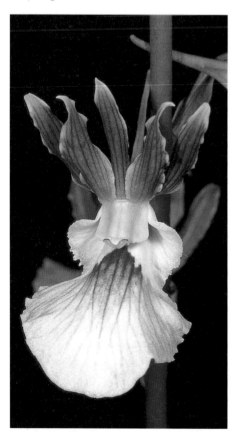

Habenaria

This genus contains over 500 species of terrestrial orchids, with tubers or fleshy roots, found throughout the tropics and subtropics, with a few temperate species. Most occur in tropical Africa but only a few are in cultivation. They need a freely drained, open compost and must be kept almost dry while dormant, although a sprinkling of water every few weeks helps to keep tubers from shrivelling. Young shoots are susceptible to rot, so care is needed in watering when growth starts in spring. All seem to be happy in intermediate conditions, in light to moderate shade.

H. procera

is a West African species that is unusual in the genus in that it is usually epiphytic in the wild. The roots are fleshy and some may break off during repotting. These can be used for propagation as they have a growing point at one end. It has a leafy stem and many long-spurred, green and white flowers in summer. Grow in a fine bark mix.

H. rhodocheila

is a striking species from China, Indochina and Malaysia. The spike bears up to 15 flowers; the sepals and petals are green but the three-lobed lip, the largest part of the flower, is yellow, orange or bright red and up to 3cm (1in) long.

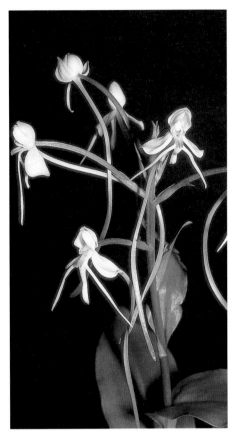

Habenaria procera

Habenaria rhodocheila

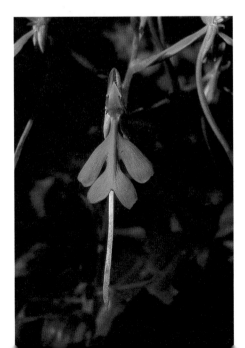

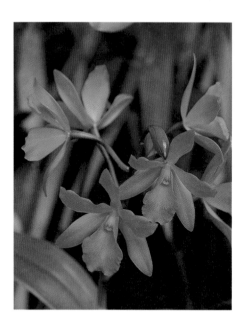

Laeliocattleya Eva

Jumellea

There are over 50 species of *Jumellea* in Madagascar and the other Indian Ocean islands, with two species on mainland Africa. The stem can be long or short, often branched at the base so that the plants form large clumps, with the leaves usually in two rows. The flowers have long spurs, are white, turning apricot as they age, and are scented in the evening. Although the flowers are borne singly, the effect of a plant scattered with starry, white flowers is beautiful. Grow in intermediate conditions, in moderate shade with high humidity, potted in a medium bark mix.

J. filicornoides
is one of the two African species. The stem can grow up to 30cm (12in) long but is often less, with two rows of dark green leaves and violet-scented white flowers.

J. fragrans
is a species that forms good clumps. The vanilla-scented leaves are used to make a herbal tea.

J. sagittata
has a short stem with several bright, glossy green leaves forming a fan. The flowers are strongly scented after dark, about 8cm (3in) in diameter, with a long spur.

Laelia

There are about 70 species of *Laelia* in Central and South America. They are very closely related to *Cattleya* and many crosses have been made between the two genera. *Laelia* species have single-leafed or two-leaved pseudobulbs, varying in shape from almost globose to cylindrical or club-shaped. The flowers are showy, in many colours – white, pink, mauve, purple, red, orange and yellow - with spreading sepals and petals and a three-lobed lip. The side lobes are often

Jumellea sagittata

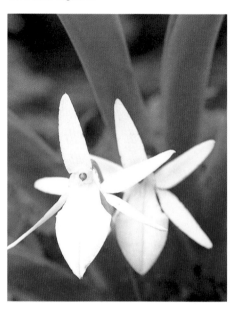

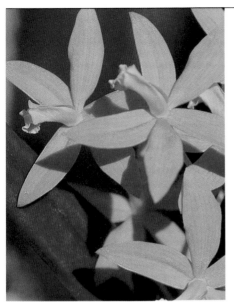

Laelia harpophylla

folded over the column so that the lip is trumpet shaped. Most species like intermediate temperatures and good light, with plenty of water and feeding in the growing season, but they need a cool, dry, bright rest in winter to encourage flowering. Many of the Brazilian species are dwarf plants that grow on rocks (often called rupicolous laelias) and a dry winter rest is important for them. They should be given only enough water to prevent the pseudobulbs shrivelling.

L. anceps
has a tall spike with scented white, pink or magenta flowers in winter.

L. autumnalis
has scented, rose-purple flowers with white or yellow on the lip, in autumn. *L. gouldiana* is very similar but flowers in summer.

L. crispa
has white flowers with a purple lip in autumn. *L. lobata* is similar.

L. flava
is a rock-growing species from Brazil with small, ovoid pseudobulbs and clusters of bright yellow flowers in spring or early summer.

L. harpophylla
has tall, slender pseudobulbs and clusters of bright orange flowers in spring. *L. cinnabarina* is similar but less slender with a taller spike of red flowers in spring to early summer.

L. pumila
is a dwarf plant with large, rose-purple flowers in spring or autumn. The lip has a frilly edge, with deep purple and yellow in the throat. It needs more shade than other species.

L. purpurata
is the National Flower of Brazil. It has large and showy flowers, 15–20cm (6–8in) in diameter, usually white or pale pink with a purple lip, but many other colour forms exist. The flowers appear in spring to summer. *L. tenebrosa* is similar but the flowers have copper-bronze sepals and petals and a purple lip.

L. sincorana
is a dwarf, rock-growing species from Brazil with showy, purple flowers.

L. speciosa,
from Mexico, is another dwarf plant with lilac-rose flowers in spring.

Ludisia

Ludisia contains one species of terrestrial orchid from China and South East Asia. This is the most common and easily grown of the jewel orchids, grown for the beauty of their leaves rather than their flowers.

L. discolor
(synonym *Haemaria discolor*) The stem is fleshy, either creeping or erect, and roots at the nodes. The leaves are evergreen, ovate and dark red-brown with red veins, although other colour forms are known. The white or yellow flowers

borne on spikes up to 30cm (12in) tall. This species grows easily in a shallow pan at intermediate or warm temperatures, in shade and with high humidity; it is a good houseplant. It can be grown in a standard houseplant compost with fine bark and perlite mixed in to give free drainage.

Miltoniopsis

These are the pansy orchids. There are five species in Central and South America with large and showy, flat-faced flowers in pink, white or pale yellow. Grow them in a fine bark compost in shade with high humidity.

M. phalaenopsis

is a white-flowered Colombian species with the lip blotched and streaked with red and purple. Flowers are borne in late spring.

Miltoniopsis Robert Strauss

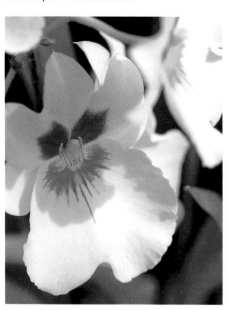

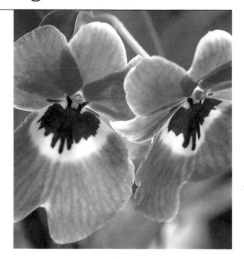

Miltoniopsis Beall's Strawberry Joy

M. vexillaria

has white or pale pink flowers in spring. The lip is yellow at the base and streaked with deep pink.

Hybrids

Pansy orchids are popular with growers for their large, long-lasting, scented flowers. The numerous hybrids are have larger flowers than the species and plants tend to be more vigorous. They do well as houseplants provided the humidity can be kept high; if they are too dry, the new leaves, when they appear, are folded in a zigzag.

Alexandre Dumas yellow flowers with red centres.

Anjou mainly deep red with white on the lip; there are several awarded clones including 'St. Patrick', AM/AOS.

Beall's Strawberry Joy pink flowers with a red and white mask.

Celle 'Wasserfal' deep purple-red flowers, the lip streaked and spotted with white giving a waterfall effect.

Emotion the various clones have white, pink or lavender flowers.

Hamburg 'Dark Tower' deep red flowers, some yellow on the lip.

Jean Carlson deep pink flowers with an orange and yellow mask.

Red Tide large red flowers.
Santa Barbara 'Rainbow Swirl' white flowers flushed with pink.
St. Helier pink flowers with a white edge; maroon-red mask.
Zorro 'Yellow Delight' primrose yellow flowers with a dark mask.

Mystacidium

This genus contains seven to ten species of small epiphytes from South Africa and eastern tropical Africa, rather like small species of *Aerangis* with spurred white or greenish-yellow flowers. All species thrive much better mounted on bark than in a pot.

M. capense,
native to South Africa and Swaziland, is the most widely grown species. It is a pretty and free-flowering plant with dark green leaves and several pendent spikes each with up to 14 starry white flowers arranged in 2 rows. It needs good light and a dryish rest in winter to stimulate flowering, which should occur in late spring or early summer.

M. venosum
is similar to *M. capense* but usually slightly smaller. It flowers in autumn and early winter and likes light to moderate shade.

Oncidium

This large genus contains about 500 species in tropical and subtropical America and is closely related to *Odontoglossum*. They vary from very small to very large plants, with large or small pseudobulbs and flowers, often on tall, branched sprays. Many are brightly coloured, usually yellow, with a prominent and often lobed lip. Most like good light and grow at intermediate temperatures. They are usually potted in a standard compost but very small species tend to do better mounted on bark.

O. cheirophorum
is a small species from Central America and Colombia with long, branching sprays of many scented, yellow flowers about 2.5cm (1in) in diameter, in summer.

O. cavendishianum
has small pseudobulbs each with one thick leaf usually described as being shaped like a mule's ear. The flowers are bright yellow, spotted with red-brown. *O. carthagense* is similar, with cream flowers spotted with magenta. Flowers are borne in summer.

O. crispum
has large flower sprays in summer, erect at first but bending over with the weight of the brown and gold flowers, which have wavy-edged petals

Mystacidium capense

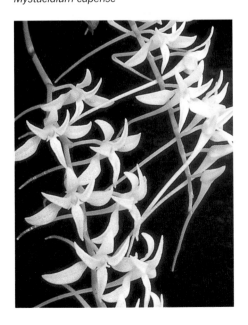

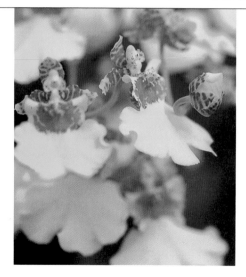

Oncidium Bois 'Sonja'.

O. maculatum
has many scented, pale yellow flowers with brown spots; the lip has a red crest.
O. pulchellum
See *Tolumnia pulchella*.
O. tigrinum
is a Mexican species with large, flat pseudobulbs and an unbranched spike growing to 40cm (16in) long. The yellow winter flowers have red-brown

Oncidium cheirophorum

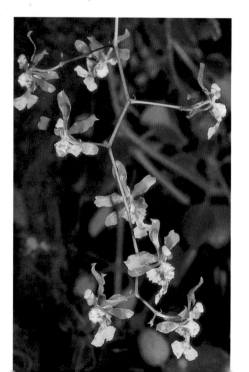

bars on the sepals and petals.
O. variegatum
See *Tolumnia variegata*, page 110.
Sharry Baby a famous hybrid with red flowers with white on the lip. 'Sweet Fragrance' is chocolate-scented.

Oncidioda
(Cochlioda x Oncidium)

These hybrids have multicoloured flowers with narrow sepals and petals.
Charlesworthii Branched spikes with many small red flowers with a pink and yellow lip.

Ornithophora

This genus contains two species of dwarf epiphyte from Brazil with pseudobulbs set well apart on the stem. Because of this spreading habit, they are better in a small basket than in a pot; they like good light and plenty of air movement.
O. radicans
(synonym *Sigmatostalix radicans*) An attractive and reliable little plant with lots of small white flowers with a maroon column and yellow anther cap, in late summer.

Paphiopedilum

Slipper orchids have always fascinated growers and their popularity is steadily increasing, not least because of some spectacular new discoveries in recent years. About 70 species are known from South East Asia, from India to the Pacific Islands; most are terrestrial but some are epiphytic or grow on rocks. Although they are sympodial orchids, they do not have pseudobulbs. The leaves are plain green or mottled,

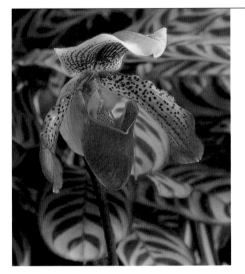

Paphiopedilum Kitty

the latter often purple below.

In most species the flowers are borne singly but in some, there are several flowers on a spike; in that case, the flowers may open all at once or in succession. All have large flowers with the characteristic pouched lip. The petals are spreading or pendulous, sometimes twisted or with hairy warts along the edges.

All paphiopedilums need a free-draining compost – more die from a soggy medium than from any other cause. But as they have no storage organs, they should not remain dry for any length of time and benefit from being repotted every year. A great variety of composts can be used; all growers seem to have their own favourites. Many find rockwool successful, in particular a mix of absorbent rockwool and horticultural foam or coarse perlite. Another widely used mix is three parts of medium bark, one part of peat or peat substitute, one part of coarse perlite, with about half a teaspoon of dolomitic limestone added. Others include a mixture of equal parts of medium and fine bark with ten per cent perlite; and a mixture of medium and fine bark with chopped sphagnum moss.

Humidity should be high and ventilation good. Almost all species grow in an intermediate greenhouse and many do well as windowsill plants or under lights. They like moderate shade although the species with plain green leaves prefer brighter light and slightly more warmth than those with mottled leaves.

P. armeniacum
is a striking Chinese species with mottled leaves and bright golden yellow flowers in spring.

P. barbatum
has mottled leaves and mainly deep purple flowers with white, purple and green stripes in winter and spring. *P. callosum* is similar but with blue-green leaves and larger, lighter flowers with downswept petals, in early summer.

P. delenatii
has attractive, mottled leaves and pale pink flowers with a deeper pink lip in spring. It comes from Vietnam and is one of the few slipper orchids that grow on acidic soils in the wild.

Paphiopedilum Magic Lantern

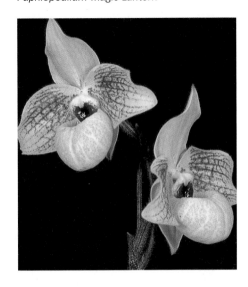

P. insigne

has plain green leaves and brownish-yellow winter flowers with green and white markings. The variety *sanderae* is green-gold with a white-edged, unspotted dorsal sepal. *P. gratrixianum* is rather similar but the leaves are longer and purple-spotted at the base; the flowers are slightly smaller with fewer dark spots on the dorsal sepal.

P. malipoense

has mottled leaves and a tall flower spike, to 30cm (12in) in height, with unusual raspberry-scented, green flowers veined with purple, in spring. It is a Chinese species, first discovered in 1984.

P. rothschildianum

is one of the finest species with a tall spike of two to five flowers, all open at once, in early summer. The sepals and petals are green-white with purple stripes, the pouch purplish; the petals have a horizontal spread of up to 30cm (12in). In the wild, it is known only from Mount Kinabalu in Borneo, but it is well established in cultivation.

P. victoria-reginae

(also known as *P. chamberlainianum*) is another multi-flowered species, from Sumatra, but the flowers open in succession and not all together. The sepals and twisted petals are green or white, streaked and blotched with purple. The pouch is purple-pink. *P. primulinum*, another Sumatran species, is similar but with slightly smaller, pale yellow flowers.

Hybrids

Over 400 hybrids were known by 1900; now over 10,000 are registered, more than in any other genus. The earliest known hybrid was Harrisianum which first flowered in 1869. *P.* Maudiae (*P. callosum* x *P. lawrenceanum*) was an early and influential hybrid with a green and white flower. 'Magnificum' and 'The Queen' are good cultivars. The breeding of hybrids has the aim of producing single, large flowers that are almost circular in shape with clear colours. White-flowered hybrids include Astarte, F.C. Puddle, Knight's Chalice, Miller's Daughter, Psyche, Shadowfax, White Knight and White Queen. Reds include Dragon Blood and Vintner's Treasure. Royale 'Downland', AM/RHS, has rose pink flowers shaded with green. Winston Churchill has mahogany red and white flowers spotted with red.

Novelty hybrids

These involve a much wider range of species. They are often multi-flowered and need not be circular in shape.

Paphiopedilum Helios

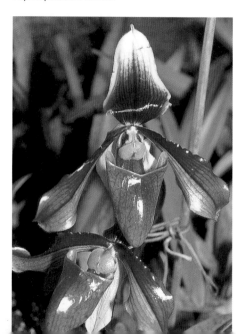

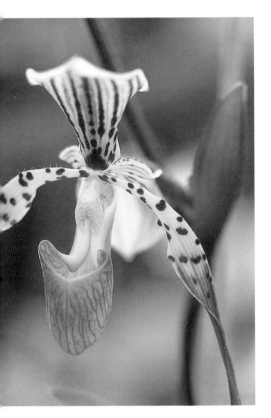

Paphiopedilum Lebaudyanum

Kevin Porter deep pink to red flowers, often with darker chequering.
Lake Shinsei deep yellow flowers.
Lynleigh Koopowitz mainly pink flowers with a mulberry scent.
Magic Lantern pink flowers.
Pearl produces many white flowers together.
Wood Dove large, red-brown flowers.
Yellow Tiger mainly yellow flowers with striped sepals and long petals.

P. rothschildianum hybrids

Some of the best hybrids have involved *P. rothschildianum*; they include:
Delrosi a succession of pink flowers.
St. Swithin white flowers, striped brown with narrow, drooping petals.
Transvaal green and white sepals and spotted and twisted petals; the pouch is pink and yellow.
Vanguard rather similar to Transvaal.

Phalaenopsis

The moth orchids include about 50 species of monopodial epiphytic orchids from Asia and Australasia with short stems and thick, usually somewhat flattened, roots. The leaves are plain green or mottled, sometimes large. The flower spike is simple or branched with showy, flat flowers. The lip of the flower has two horn-like projections at the apex.

Grow *Phalaenopsis* in pots or baskets in a coarse bark mix, in moderate to heavy shade with high humidity, at intermediate to warm temperatures. Water should not be allowed to lodge in the

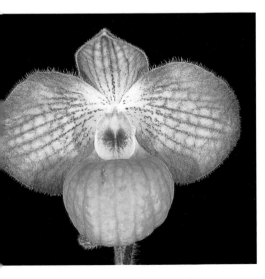

Paphiopedilum Lynleigh Koopowitz

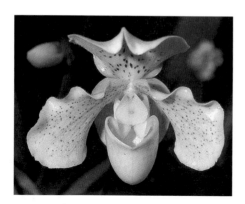

Paphiopedilum Silberhorn

centre of the plant overnight as this causes rot. Do not be in a hurry to cut off old flower stalks; while they remain green they may branch and flower again. Sometimes keikis are produced on the spike instead of flowers; these can be removed and potted up once they have grown roots. The moth orchids are currently among the most popular of all orchids, widely sold as houseplants. The flowers are long-lasting and they adapt well to windowsill culture, as long as they do not get direct sun. An almost limitless range of hybrids is available, with white, pink or yellow flowers, often striped with another colour.

P. amabilis
(synonym *P. grandiflora*) has glossy, dark green leaves and scented, white, often pink-tinged flowers, the lip with red and yellow marks. This winter-flowering species is in the ancestry of most modern hybrids.

P. equestris
has dark green leaves, often purple below, and arching sprays of many pink flowers around 4cm (1½in) in diameter.

P. mannii
is compact, with dark green leaves and yellow flowers barred with brown.

P. schilleriana,
from the Philippines, has lovely dark green leaves mottled with silver, and branched, many-flowered sprays of white, pink, mauve or purple flowers, mostly in winter. *P. stuartiana*, another Philippine species, has similar leaves and white flowers with the sepals spotted with red-brown at the base.

Hybrids
These are attractive to commercial growers as they can reach flowering size in less than three years from seed. Many are propagated by tissue culture. New hybrids are constantly being registered. They tend to be similar in the shape of the flower, the differences being mainly in colour. Hybrids with *P. equestris* in their ancestry have smaller flowers, but more of them. Hybrids of *P. schilleriana* have beautifully mottled leaves. The following is a very small selection of what is available.

WHITE
Allegria
Capitola 'Moonlight'
Doris
Gladys Read 'Snow Queen'
Happy Girl (white with a red lip)
Henriette Lecoufle 'Boule de Neige'

Phalaenopsis 'Golden Horizon Sunrise'

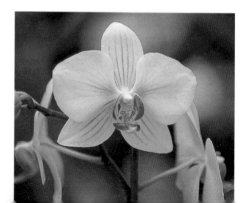

Mini Mark 'Maria Theresa', AAM/AOS (white with orange spots and an orange lip)
Opaline
Red Fan (white with a red lip)

PINK
Formosa Rose
Hilo Lip (pink with a white lip)
Hokuspocus
Lippeglut (dark pink lip)
Lipperose (dark pink lip)
Little Mary (dark pink lip)
Mistinguette (dotted with darker pink)
Party Dress
Patea 'Hawaii' (deep pink)
Romance
Sourire (pale to deep pink with mottled leaves)

YELLOW
Golden Amboin (spotted with brown)
Golden Buddha
Golden Emperor
Gorey 'Trinity'
Orchid World
Orglade's Lemon Dew
Sierra Gold 'Suzanne', FCC/AOS

RED
Cordova 'Ken's Ruby'
Ember 'East Red' (magenta)
Firelight 'Stone's River' (magenta)
Sophie Hausermann
Summer Morn 'Shari Mowlavi', AM/AOS

STRIPED
Hennessy (white or pink with red or pink stripes)
Modest Girl (white with pink stripes)
Nero Wolf (pink stripes with a darker pink, red lip)
Zuma Chorus (pink stripes on magenta)

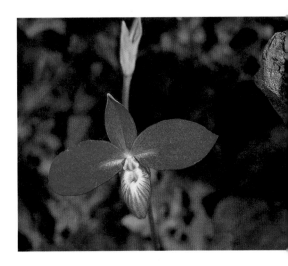

Phragmipedium besseae

Phragmipedium

The South American slipper orchids are less widely cultivated than their Asiatic relatives, *Paphiopedilum*, but their popularity has increased in recent years. There are about 20 species in Central and South America that differ only in botanical detail from *Paphiopedilum*. Much of the current interest was stimulated by the discovery of the red-flowered *P. besseae* in Peru in 1981, followed in 1987 by the discovery of another form of the same species in Ecuador, and their subsequent use in hybridization.

They require similar conditions to *Paphiopedilum*, except that they seem to need more frequent watering. They should not be divided too often as they do better in big clumps.

P. besseae
has bright scarlet flowers about 6cm (2½in) in diameter. The variety *dalessandroi*, the form from Ecuador, has a more branched flower spike with more numerous, but slightly smaller, flowers

that are usually orange-red. Flowers appear in autumn.

P. longifolium

has a tall flower spike with several flowers opening over a long period. The flowers are yellow-green, the petals edged with purple, the lip with purple spots. It flowers off and on throughout the year.

P. pearcei

is a dwarf species from Ecuador and Peru, where it often grows on boulders in rivers. It has narrow, dark green leaves and green and purple flowers about 7.5cm (3in) in diameter, with ribbon-like, twisted petals.

P. schlimii

is a Colombian species with a branched or unbranched flower spike to 50cm (20in) high, with pink and white flowers.

Hybrids

Don Wimber very large orange flowers, produced freely.

Elizabeth March pink and white flowers .

Eric Young large, salmon to orange flowers.

Hanne Popow the first *P. besseae* hybrid to be registered, in 1992; the colour ranges from apricot to pale pink and deep pink.

Mem. Dick Clements a relatively compact plant with many deep red flowers. Other good reds include Living Fire, Ruby Slippers and Jason Fischer.

Sedenii an old hybrid made over 100 years ago with long-lasting pink and white flowers opening off and on for most of the year.

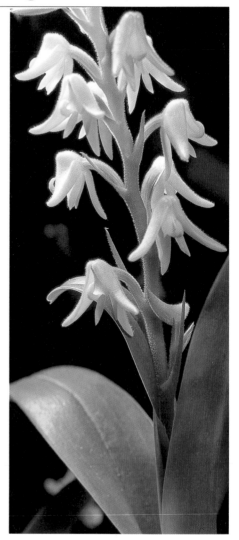

Polystachya bella

Polystachya

There are about 200 species of *Polystachya* found throughout the tropics but with most in Africa. They are small to medium plants, almost all epiphytic, with pseudobulbs varying from small and round to flat and coin-like or narrowly cylindrical. The long-lasting flowers are usually small with the lip held uppermost, in a range of colours; most are scented. Plants can be mounted on bark if the humidity is high enough, or potted in a fine bark mix that should be allowed to dry out between waterings.

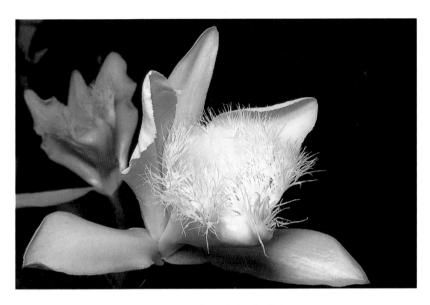

Rhyncholaelia digbyana

P. bella

is a lovely species with golden yellow to orange flowers, known only from one area in Kenya but well established in cultivation. The pseudobulbs grow on an ascending stem so plants in pots should be given a branch or a moss pole to climb. It flowers off and on through the year.

P. campyloglossa

has very strongly and sweetly scented lime-green to yellow-green flowers with a white lip.

P. cultriformis

has conical, single-leafed pseudobulbs and branched spikes of numerous flowers in white, yellow or pale to deep pink.

P. fallax

is another very fragrant species with white and yellow flowers off and on throughout the year.

P. rosea

is a relatively tall species from Madagascar with an erect, branched flower spike up to 30cm (12in) high; the pink flowers are small but numerous.

Rhyncholaelia

A genus with two species of epiphytic orchid from Mexico and Central America, formerly included in *Brassavola*.

R. digbyana

(synonym *Brassavola digbyana*) has club-shaped pseudobulbs each with one stiff, grey-green leaf. The large, long-lasting flowers are scented, usually yellow-green; the lip is white or cream tinged with green, and the mid lobe is deeply fringed. Grow potted in a coarse mix in bright light.

Stanhopea

About 25 species of large epiphytic orchids from tropical America, with smallish pseudobulbs, each with one large, pleated leaf. The flowers are large, strangely shaped and strongly scented, but last for only two or three days. Because the flower spikes grow downwards, stanhopeas must be grown in baskets in a coarse bark mix. They like good light, a humid atmosphere and plenty of water while in growth.

S. oculata
has creamy yellow flowers with red blotches on each side of the lip base, in summer.
S. tigrinum
has bright orange flowers blotched with maroon-red.
S. wardii
has yellow flowers; the lip is orange with deep red-black eye spots on either side of the base.

Stanhopea oculata

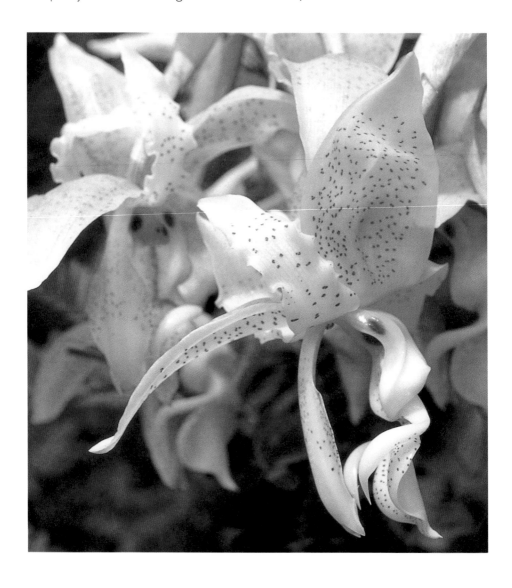

Vanilla

A genus with about 100 species of scrambling and climbing orchids found throughout the tropics. The stems are green, stout and fleshy, with many roots. Some cling (like ivy) and some grow down until they reach the ground. Some species have large, fleshy leaves while others have only scale leaves and appear leafless. The flowers are large, usually with spreading sepals and petals and a trumpet-shaped lip, but are not usually produced until the plant has reached a considerable height. Plant in pots in a standard bark mix, with a long moss pole for the stem to climb – it should be tied to the pole to start with. When the top of the pole is reached, the stem can either be allowed to dangle (which sometimes stimulates flowering) or be trained horizontally along a pole parallel to the ridge of the greenhouse or conservatory. Even when not in flower, the plants look interesting.

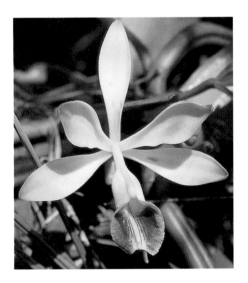

Vanilla polylepis

V. planifolia
is the commercial vanilla, native to Central America and the West Indies but widely planted and often naturalized elsewhere, particularly in Madagascar. The capsules are still used to produce vanilla flavouring, far superior to synthetic vanilla essence. The flowers are yellow-green, about 10cm (4in) in diameter. There is a form with variegated leaves.

V. pompona
(synonym *V. grandiflora*) has leaves up to 25cm (10in) long and yellow-green flowers about 15cm (6in) in diameter with orange marks on the lip.

V. polylepis
is a tropical African species with very attractive flowers, white or greenish-white. The lip has a yellow blotch in the throat and is usually maroon-purple towards the apex.

The following orchids can be grown in the warmer parts of an intermediate greenhouse, but they will grow and flower better in a warm house.

Orchids for the warm greenhouse

minimum night-time temperature **18°C(65°F)**

9

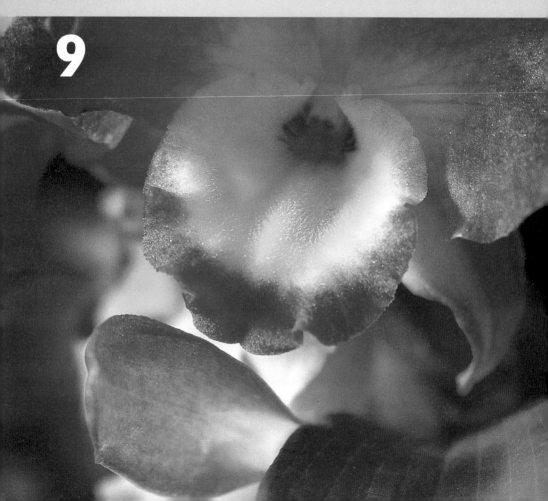

Orchids for the warm greenhouse

Aerides

This genus includes about 20 species of monopodial epiphytes from Asia with showy spikes of scented flowers, usually white, pink or purplish. They are large plants that like warm, humid conditions so in spite of their striking display, they are not often grown in Europe. They have many long, aerial roots and do well in baskets.

A. multiflora

(synonym *A. affinis*) is a robust plant with leaves up to 30cm (12in) long, and large sprays of white or pink flowers in summer.

A. rosea

(synonym *A. fieldingii*) is similar to *A. multiflora* but with slightly larger purple flowers, tinged with white, in dense spikes up to 35cm (14in) long, which appear in summer.

Angraecum

Some species of *Angraecum* grow best in a warm greenhouse, although they will grow in the warmer parts of an intermediate house (see page 77).

A. eburneum

is a large, robust species with several pairs of leathery, strap-shaped leaves. The flower spikes are erect with up to 30 flowers with green sepals and petals and a white, shell-shaped lip which is held uppermost. There are four subspecies from different geographical areas that differ slightly in size and proportions of lip. Subspecies *superbum* is the largest and its variety *longicalcar* has probably the longest spur known in any orchid – up to 35cm (14in) long. *A. eburneum* likes good light; it is a striking plant, but large.

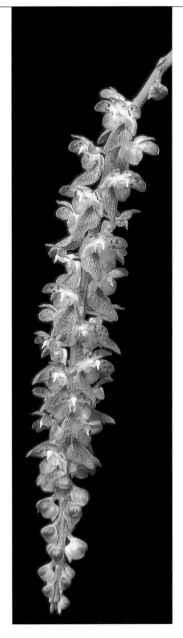

Aerides multiflora

Ascocentrum

This genus contains five species of epiphytic orchid resembling small vandas, occurring in Asia from India to the Philippines. The stems are erect, with two rows of leaves; the brightly coloured red, orange or pink flowers are in dense, erect spikes. Grow in pots or baskets in a medium to coarse bark mix or mounted on a slab. They like good light and high humidity and regular feeding and watering while in growth; keep drier in winter. They will grow in the warmer parts of an intermediate house, but are better in a warm house.

A. ampullaceum

is a compact species with bright cherry-pink flowers in spring. The variety *aurantiacum* has orange flowers.

A. curvifolium

is larger, with stems to 25cm (10in) long. The flowers are deep orange to red with a yellow lip and a purple column. An attractive species which has been widely used in hybridization.

A. garayi

has bright golden-orange flowers very freely borne.

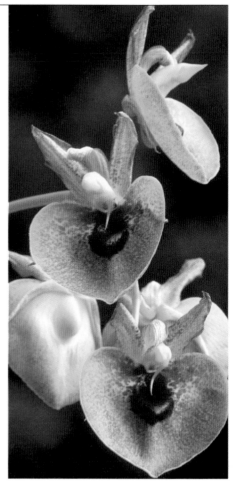

Catasetum expansum

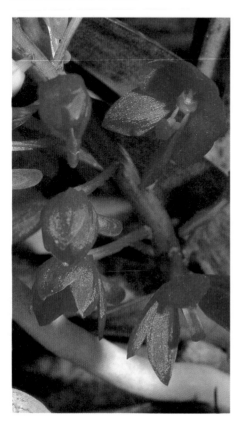

Ascocentrum ampullaceum

Catasetum

These are sympodial orchids, most epiphytic, from tropical Central and South America and the West Indies. Estimates of the number of species vary from 50 to 130. They are unusual among orchids in that the flowers are either male or female, usually carried on different plants but sometimes on the same plant. They often look very different; the male flowers are usually brightly coloured and the female flowers are usually yellow-green. All have fleshy pseudobulbs and large, pleated leaves, usually deciduous in winter. The flower spikes may be erect, arching or pendent. Grow in pots or baskets in a coarse bark compost, at intermediate or warm temperatures and in bright light. Give plenty of water and fertilizer while growing but in winter give only enough water to stop the pseudo-bulbs from shrivelling. Humidity should be high while plants are growing actively.

C. barbatum
usually has green male flowers with maroon spots and a hair-fringed lip. The female flowers are similar but smaller, without the fringe on the lip. Flowers appear in summer.

C. saccatum
is a variable species from Brazil, Peru and Guyana. The male flowers can be white, green, purple-brown, orange or purple; the female flowers are yellow-green. Flowers are borne in summer.

C. tenebrosum
has male flowers with maroon-brown sepals and a fleshy lip in yellow, lime green or purple. The female flowers are greenish-red. Flowers appear in summer.

Hybrids
Some fine *Catasetum* hybrids have been registered in recent years but few are widely available.

Orchidglade has yellow-green flowers very heavily mottled with maroon.

Dendrobium

Some species of *Dendrobium* need warm conditions throughout the year and although they, too, should be kept drier when not in active growth they should not remain dry for long periods. They can make good houseplants and seem to be particularly successful in a kitchen with an Aga or Rayburn cooker, which is always warm.

D. bigibbum
(synonym *D. phalaenopsis*) has stout, upright canes and arching spikes of about 20 white, lilac or pink flowers with a darker lip. It is found in New Guinea and Australia. Large-flowered forms were known as *D. phalaenopsis* but are now usually treated as *D. bigibbum* subsp. *phalaenopsis*. Many beautiful hybrids have been developed from this species and are important in East Asia for the cut-flower trade.

American Beauty magenta-purple flowers.

Bangkok Fancy lavender to purple flowers.

Dendrobium Thai Fancy

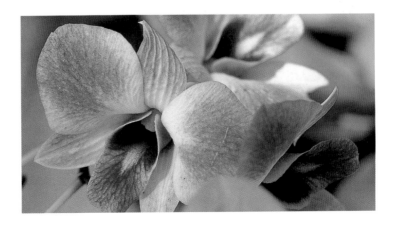

Candy Stripe pale pink flowers with deeper pink stripes.
Dale Takiguchi white flowers.
Doreen 'Kodama' white flowers.
Lady Fay magenta-purple flowers.
Lady Hamilton magenta-purple flowers.
Orglade's Orbit - magenta-purple flowers.

Doritis

There are two or three species of *Doritis* in East Asia; they are closely related to *Phalaenopsis*. These plants have short stems, stiff fleshy leaves, thick flattened roots and showy flowers. They grow well in pots or baskets with a medium bark compost and require plenty of water and fertilizer while in growth; even when resting, they should not dry out completely. *Doritis* species are grown less often than *Doritaenopsis*, their hybrids with *Phalaenopsis*

D. pulcherrima

(synonym *D. esmeralda*) has a large flower spike, up to 60cm (24in) tall in summer; the numerous flowers are usually magenta but sometimes paler. The variety *coerulea* has blue-violet flowers.

Doritis pulcherrima

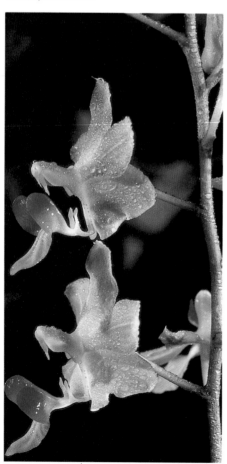

Doritaenopsis
(Doritis x Phalaenopsis)

These are vigorous, free-flowering plants with characteristics halfway between the parents. The long-lasting flowers are white, pink or red, usually spotted or striped with a darker colour. The flowers appear on tall, often branched, spikes usually in summer.
Coral Gleam deep pink flowers.
Flame Mountain 'Zuma Boy' deep pink with red stripes.
George Moler white flowers striped with pink and a deep red lip.
Happy Valentine large pink flowers with a red or orange lip.
Krull's Dazzler 'Ponkans Cherries Jubilee', AM/AOS deep pink flowers with a darker lip.
Lady Jewel white flowers.
Orglade's Puff white flowers with gold marks on the lip.
Purple Gem 'Vivid' bright magenta flowers.
Red Coral deep pinkish-red flowers on branched stems.

Euanthe

This genus includes one species of monopodial epiphyte from the Philippines, formerly included in *Vanda*.

E. sanderiana

(synonyms *Esmeralda sanderiana* and *Vanda sanderiana*) is a beautiful species with a tall, leafy stem with flower spikes arising from the leaf axils. The flat-faced flowers are 10cm (4in) in diameter and are pale to deep pink, with the lower half of the flower veined and streaked with purple-brown. Grow in a pot or basket in a coarse bark mix in good light, with plenty of water and feeding while in active growth but less in winter.

Psychopsis

These are the butterfly orchids. The genus includes about five species of epiphytes from Central and South America,

Psychopsis papilio

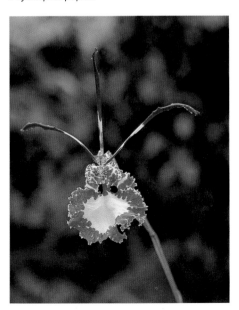

sometimes included in *Oncidium*, with clustered, single-leafed pseudobulbs and often mottled leaves. The erect or arching flower spikes bear showy flowers with a narrow, erect dorsal sepal and petals resembling antennae. The frilly lip is yellow and brown. Do not cut off old flower spikes even if they look as they have finished, because flowers may still be produced. Grow in a very open, coarse compost or mounted, in warm, shady, humid conditions.

P. papilio (synonym *Oncidium papilio* and *Oncidium picta*) has tall spikes, up to 1m (3ft) high or even more, each with many flowers. The yellow and brown striped flowers open one or two at a time over a long period.

Rhynchostylis

These are the foxtail orchids. The genus includes about six species of monopodial epiphytes from Asia. Stems are short, the roots long and numerous and the leaves thick and leathery. The flower spikes are usually pendent and cylindrical and bear many flowers. The flowers are white or pink, with purple markings. Because of their long roots and pendent spikes this species should be grown in baskets in a coarse, free-draining compost.

R. gigantea

has spikes up to 35cm (14in) long. The waxy flowers are about 3cm (1in) in diameter, usually white spotted with violet and purple, but pure white and rose-purple forms are known.

R. retusa

has flower spikes up to 45cm (18in) long, bearing small white flowers, spotted with pink and violet.

Tolumnia

Tolumnia includes about 20 species of small epiphyte from Central America and the West Indies, closely related to *Oncidium* and still usually referred to as the 'equitant' or 'variegata' oncidiums. They have no pseudobulbs and the leaves form a fan. The flowers are big for the size of plant with a large, usually four-lobed lip. It is best to mount the plants, as they rot easily if water lodges among the leaves, but with careful watering they can be grown in small pots in a very free-draining compost. They like good light, good air movement and high humidity.

T. pulchella
(synonym *Oncidium pulchellum*) has an arched spike bearing many white, pink or magenta flowers.

T. variegata
(synonym *Oncidium variegatum*) is slightly smaller with white or pink flowers marked with brown or crimson.

Vanda

This genus contains about 40 species of monopodial orchids from tropical Asia. The stems are usually long and leafy, with roots along their length and flower spikes arising in the leaf joints. The flat-faced flowers are showy. Plants are usually grown in baskets in a coarse, bark-based compost but in the Far East, where vandas are widely grown, they are often grown in baskets with no compost at all, the roots attaching themselves to the basket or hanging free. They like bright light and most prefer warm, or warm to intermediate temperatures.

V. coerulea
has a stem up to 1.5m (5ft) long. The flowers are about 10cm (4in) in diameter and pale to deep lilac-blue. This species comes from higher altitudes than most and can be grown in a cool greenhouse as it dislikes high winter temperatures. It flowers in autumn to winter.

V. coerulescens
is a much smaller plant than the last with the stem only about 10cm (4in) long. The flowers are 4cm (11/2in) in diameter, blue-violet with a darker lip.

V. tricolor
(synonym *V. suavis*) has a stem up to 1m (3ft) tall. The flowers are scented, 8cm (3in) in diameter and usually white or pale yellow spotted with red-brown. The lip is magenta and white. Flowers appear in autumn and winter.

Hybrids

Many beautiful hybrids are available but because of their size and their need for high temperatures, they are much more widely grown in the Far East than in Europe or most of America. There are many hybrids with *Ascocentrum* – see *Ascocenda* (page 79).

Vanda Miss Joachim a tall plant with cylindrical leaves and lavender flowers with a large, dark rose pink lip.

Vanda Rothschildiana a compact but vigorous plant with large, deep lavender blue flowers with darker chequering, appearing in winter.

Vanda Rothschildiana

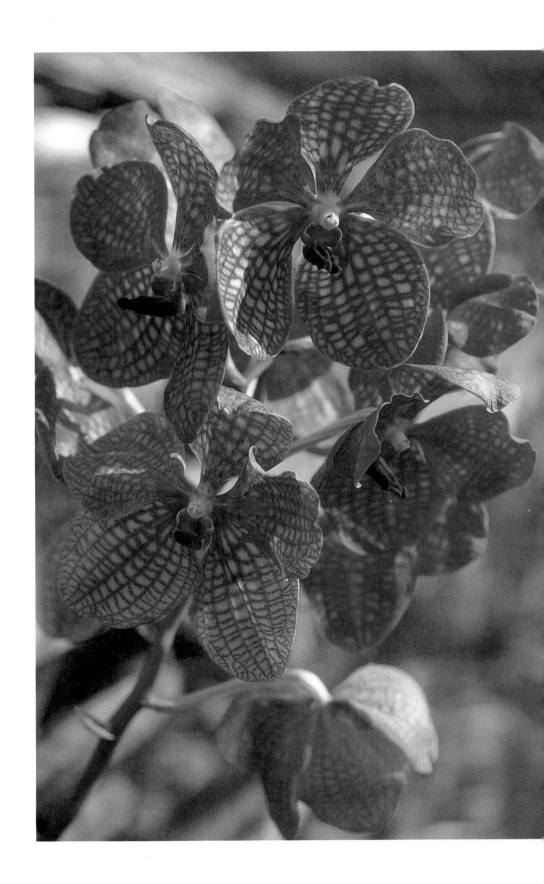

Orchids that do well in an alpine house include those that can withstand low but not freezing temperatures and also those that can survive sub-zero temperatures but dislike winter wet. All these plants also do well in an unheated conservatory.

Orchids for the alpine house

minimum night-time temperature **0°C(32°F)**

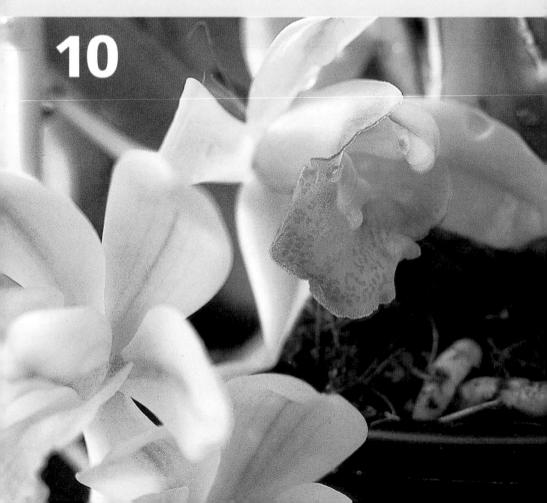

10

Bletilla

This genus includes about 10 species of terrestrial orchids from Japan and China, which are almost hardy in temperate climates. They have corm-like pseudobulbs and deciduous, pleated leaves and will grow in any well-drained, peat-based or loam-based compost if it is alkaline

B. striata

(synonym *B. hyacinthina*) is by far the most common species in cultivation, sometimes sold in garden centres. The flowers are rose-purple and grow on an erect spike that appears from between the leaves in early summer. There is a white form with a yellow throat, but this is much less easy to obtain.

Calanthe

The deciduous calanthes have already been described (see page 82). While evergreen species can be either tropical or temperate, it is the temperate ones that are more often grown. They are almost hardy and do well in alpine house conditions. They grow in any free-draining terrestrial compost and need plenty of water while in growth but should be kept drier, but not completely dry, in winter. Several are native to Japan, where they are popular plants.

C. discolor

is a spring-flowering Japanese species with a flower spike 40–50cm (16–20in) tall. The flowers are either white, pink or maroon with a pink lip.

C. reflexa

is a small, spring-flowering Japanese species with the flower spikes reaching only 15cm (6in) high. The flowers are white, pink or magenta with a darker lip and a yellow base.

Bletilla striata

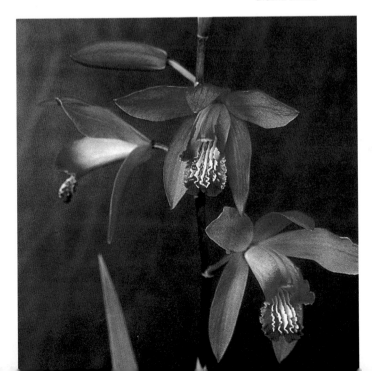

C. striata

(synonym *C. sieboldii*) is another Japanese species with the flower spikes growing up to 45cm (18in) tall, bearing large, yellow flowers in early summer.

Cymbidium

One or two species of *Cymbidium* are hardy enough to be grown out of doors in a sheltered spot, but it is safer to grow them in an alpine house or as a house plant. Use the same composts and general cultivation methods as for the other cymbidiums described in Chapter 7 (see page 55).

C. goeringii,

native to China and Japan, is believed to have been cultivated in China for over 2,000 years and in Japan for many hundreds of years. Many varieties are available there. It has dark green, grassy leaves and flowers borne singly on a stalk 10–15cm (4–6in) long. The flowers open in winter or spring and are about 5cm (2in) in diameter and sometimes scented. They are green, yellow-green, brown or brownish-orange with a white lip marked with red or purple.

Ophrys

This genus contains 30–50 species of tuberous terrestrial orchid occurring in Europe, North Africa and the Middle East, with most from the Mediterranean region. Four species are British natives. They are plants that always attract attention as the flowers mimic various female insects so effectively that the males try to mate with them and, in so doing, carry pollen from one flower to another. A few species are now available from specialist nurseries; they can be grown in the open garden but are more often grown in pots in an alpine house. Drainage must be good and most species require a hot, dry summer to do well. After flowering in spring and summer, plants die back until rosettes of leaves appear in late winter. In the wild, most species grow on chalk and limestone, so dolomitic limestone or limestone chips should be added to the compost. A recommended *Ophrys* compost is three parts of sterile loam to three parts of coarse gritty sand, two parts of sieved beech or oak leafmould and one part of fine pine bark, plus some limestone chips and a little hoof and horn fertilizer.

O. apifera

the bee orchid, is widespread in Europe. It has pink sepals and petals and a furry brown and green lip.

O. fusca

is a Mediterranean species that is supposed to be one of the easier species in cultivation. It grows 10–40cm (4–16in) tall, with green to yellow sepals, yellow to brown petals and a dark brown lip.

O. insectifera

the fly orchid is a British native, a slender plant with green sepals, black antenna-like petals and a furry dark brown lip with a blue base.

Pleione

This genus includes about 20 mainly terrestrial species found from India east to Taiwan and Thailand. They used to be known as windowsill orchids, but as so

Pleione bulbocodioides

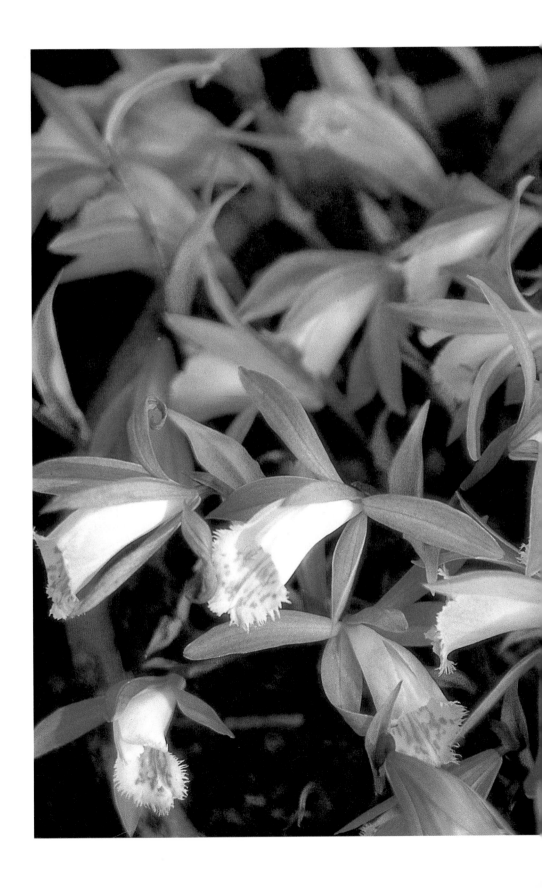

many other kinds of orchids are now grown indoors, that name is less appropriate than it was. They produce clumps of pseudobulbs, each with one or two leaves. The flowers are showy and large for the size of the plant, in white, pink, mauve or yellow, usually with darker markings on the lip.

Most species are hardy down to 0°C (32°F) and so in theory they could be grown out of doors in milder areas. They do not, however, like winter wet and are much better indoors or in an alpine house over winter, although they can be put outside in a shady, sheltered place in summer. Plant them in shallow pots, preferably terracotta. Numerous different composts are used, but as for all terrestrial orchids, the most important factor is that it is free-draining. One suitable mix consists of six parts of fine orchid bark to one part of coarse perlite or perlag, one part of chopped sphagnum moss and one part of chopped bracken fronds or chopped freshly fallen oak or beech leaves.

The pseudobulbs should be cleaned up and repotted in January or February. Trim the old roots down to about 1cm (1/2in) long and cut away any old, loose sheaths. Plant the pseudobulbs close together and just deep enough to anchor them in the compost. Keep at a temperature of 0–10°C (32–50°F) until you see the flower buds emerging, then bring indoors and start to water carefully. When the flowers are over, the leaves grow rapidly so water and a balanced fertilizer can be given freely.

In July, change to a fertilizer that is higher in phosphate and potassium to encourage flowering the following year. When the leaves turn yellow and fall, the plants should be kept dry until you repot the following January.

Two species, *P. praecox* and *P. maculata*, and a few hybrids derived from them, flower in autumn but are treated in the same way as spring-flowering plants. All the species and hybrids of *Pleione* are rather similar in general appearance, with spreading sepals and petals and a fringed, trumpet-shaped lip. The flower spike is rarely taller than 20cm (8in) and bears one or two flowers.

P. bulbocodioides

has lilac-pink to magenta flowers with purple-brown marks on the lip. There is a pretty white form.

P. x confusa

is a natural hybrid of *P. forrestii*, with larger and often paler flowers.

P. formosana

has pale or mid lilac-pink flowers, the lip paler with yellow marks. This is the most common species in cultivation and there are numerous cultivars, including 'Blush of Dawn' and 'Oriental Splendour'. 'Clare' and 'Snow White' have white flowers.

P. forrestii

has yellow flowers, the lip spotted with brown or red.

P. speciosa

has purplish pseudobulbs and bright magenta flowers; the lip has pale orange markings and yellow crests.

Hybrids

More and more hybrids are becoming available; they are often more vigorous and free-flowering than the species from which they are derived.

Alishan lilac flowers, lip white with red marks. 'Goldfinch', 'Merlin' and 'Sparrowhawk' are good cultivars.

Eiger white flowers.
El Pico mauve to deep rose-purple
flowers.
Shantung usually yellow or creamy
white flowers flushed with pink.
'Fieldfare' has large, pale yellow flowers;
'Muriel Harberd' has large, apricot
flowers.
Stromboli deep rose-purple flowers
with an orange-blotched lip. 'Fireball'
has particularly intense colouring.
Tolima mauve to deep pink flowers.
Tongariro purple flowers, marked
with red and yellow; 'Jackdaw' has the
deepest colour.
Versailles the first *Pleione* hybrid. The
flowers are pale to deep pink;
'Bucklebury' flowers very freely.

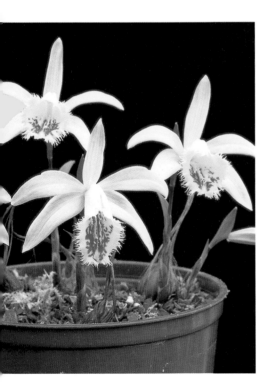

Pleione Shantung 'Ridgeway'

Pterostylis

Pterostylis includes about 80 species of
terrestrial orchids known as greenhoods;
almost all are found in Australia and
New Zealand. The flowers are green,
often tinged with purple, and the uppermost sepal is arched and forms a hood
with the petals. Some species are almost
hardy in temperate climates but do not
tolerate winter wet, so they are best
grown in an alpine house or cool greenhouse. They dislike chalk and are usually
grown in a compost mixture such as two
parts of gritty sand to one part of sterile
loam, one part of fine orchid bark and a
sprinkling of bonemeal.

Plants are dormant in summer,
the leaves appear in autumn and plants
continue to grow throughout the winter.
Some species form colonies in the wild
and increase rapidly in cultivation. After
flowering, keep the compost dry and
resume watering with care when new
growths start to appear.
P. cucullata
is a colony-forming species with
brown or brown and green flowers
in early spring.
P. curta
is a species that increases quickly.
It grows to 30cm (12in) tall and has
whitish flowers veined with green
and tinged with brown, which open
in late summer.

Quite a number of orchids are hardy
enough to be grown in temperate
gardens. Most like a well-drained
soil that does not dry out completely.
Orchids can be established in a
lawn and in fact they sometimes
establish themselves.

Orchids for
the garden
minimum night-time temperature **10°C(50°F)**

11

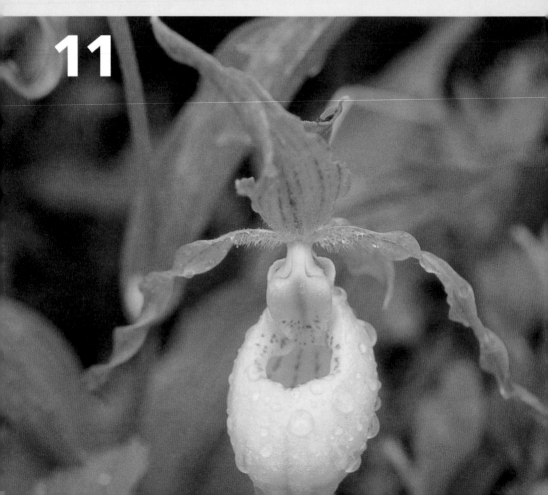

Orchids for the garden

Orchids look great in the garden, and many are relatively easy to cultivate. A wildflower meadow can be created with lesser butterfly orchids (*Platanthera bifolia*), heath spotted orchids (*Dactylorhiza maculata* subsp. *ericetorum*) and northern marsh orchids (*Dactylorhiza purpurella*), for example. On chalky soil, autumn lady's tresses (*Spiranthes spiralis*) will sometimes appear spontaneously in lawns and tennis courts. Where orchids are growing in grass, management of the grass is important as the orchids are easily choked out. The grass should be cut (or grazed) in spring before the flowers start to develop, and then left alone until the flowers have faded and the seed has been shed. Then cutting or grazing can be resumed until the following spring.

Orchids can be erratic in their appearance; they may grow in profusion one year, then for no apparant reason, in far fewer numbers the next year. Terrestrial orchids seem able to persist underground for many years. When a piece of grassland that has been over-grazed or, conversely, allowed to grow rank is properly managed once again, orchids often reappear within a couple of years.

While some of the larger species of *Dactylorhiza*, such as *D. foliosa*, the Madeira orchid, seem to enjoy a rich, border soil, most wild orchids are happier in soil of low fertility. In the past, the main obstacle to growing hardy orchids in the garden was lack of availability but now several nurseries offer seed-grown plants of an increasing range of species.

These establish much more readily than plants lifted from the wild, a practice that is, in any case, against the law in most countries. In cold areas, several of the orchids mentioned below, such as species of *Orchis*, are more satisfactory grown in an alpine house.

Cypripedium

Some species of lady's slippers can be grown in gardens. As with other species of hardy terrestrial orchids, interest is increasing and seed-grown plants are becoming more widely available.

C. acaule,
the moccasin flower, is a summer-flowering North American species with brownish sepals and petals and a deep pink lip. It can be temperamental in cultivation.

C. calceolus,
the lady's slipper orchid, is hovering on the edge of extinction in Britain but is still relatively common in other countries. It has maroon-brown (occasionally green) sepals and petals and a bright yellow lip. It does not like acid soil.

Cypripedium parviflorum var. *pubescens*

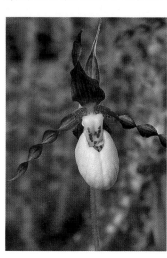

C. parviflorum

(also known as *C. calceolus* var. *parviflorum*) is the North American form of *C. calceolus* and has at times been treated as a variety of that species. The summer flowers are smaller than those of *C. calceolus* but the colouring is similar: sepals and petals are purple to maroon, the lip yellow with red spots inside. Two varieties are recognized: var. *parviflorum* and var. *pubescens*. Both grow well in gardens in a good but well-drained soil and will form good clumps when established. They are probably the easiest species of *Cypripedium* to cultivate and, unlike *C. calceolus*, will grow in acid soils.

C. reginae,

the queen lady's slipper orchid, is a very handsome North American species with white or pale pink flowers with a deeper pink lip. In the wild, it grows in bogs but in cultivation it prefers a well-drained soil. The flowers appear in summer.

Dactylorhiza

These are the easiest of the hardy orchids to grow in most gardens. There are about 40 species, many rather similar, which are widespread in Europe, extending into Asia, with one or two in North America. They are closely related to *Orchis* but differ in having tubers with finger-like projections. Most grow well in a good, well-drained garden soil, preferably in light shade, and flower in summer. More species are now becoming available from seed-grown plants and any that can be obtained are worth growing. Several hybrids are starting to appear on the market and they seem to be even more vigorous than the species.

D. elata

is a handsome species native to South West Europe and North Africa, but it seems to be hardy in almost all temperate gardens. Plants have plain green leaves and tall, dense heads of rich purple flowers in summer. They increase well to form good clumps.

D. foliosa,

the Madeira orchid, grows wild only on the island of Madeira. It is a beautiful species, very similar to *D. elata*, differing mainly in lip shape, and grows and increases well in similar situations.

D. fuchsii,

the common spotted orchid, is an attractive species that is widespread in Britain. It has spotted leaves and pale to deep lilac-pink flowers with darker spots, in late spring or early summer. It grows taller and more luxuriantly in gardens than in the wild. Although it often grows on chalk, it also grows well on neutral to slightly acid soils.

D. maculata

subsp. *ericetorum*, the heath spotted orchid, occurs on more acid soils. It is a smaller plant than *D. fuchsii* with a shorter flower spike, but is also a pretty little plant.

Dactylorhiza fuchsii

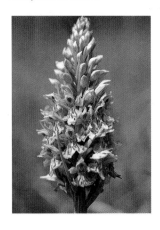

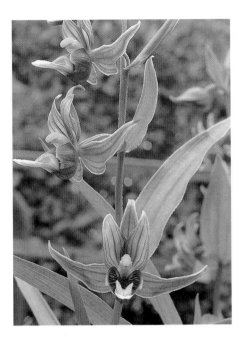

Epipactis gigantea

Epipactis

This genus includes over 20 species of terrestrial orchids, mostly temperate but a few tropical, with creeping stems and fleshy roots. The following can be grown in the open garden.

E. gigantea

is a North American species with a rather misleading name as it is not very big. The stems are leafy, 30–60cm (12–24in) tall, with yellow-brown flowers striped with pink or purple which appear in late spring and summer. It increases well in light shade, in a soil which is well drained but does not dry out completely.

E. palustris,

the marsh helleborine, is a British native similar to the last species. The sepals are purplish-brown, the petals white tinged with pink at the base, and the lip white marked with yellow. It likes a fairly damp situation, preferably not in acid soil.

Orchis

Orchis contains about 30 species of terrestrial orchid with ovoid tubers, occurring in Europe and temperate Asia, as far east as China. There are seven British native species, although most are rare. A few can be grown in an open garden, either in a rock garden or naturalized in grass. However, most growers have them in pots in an alpine house, using a similar compost to that given for *Ophrys* (see page 114).

O. mascula,

the early purple orchid, is the most common of the British species, growing 15–60cm (6–24in) tall with leaves heavily spotted with purple. The light purple flowers have darker spots and appear in dense spikes in spring.

O. laxiflora,

the lax-flowered orchid, is fairly widespread in Europe. It is a tall plant with a loose spike of rose-pink or lilac flowers in spring and early summer.

O. morio,

the green-veined orchid, used to be common in Britain but is now much rarer. It varies from 5–50cm (2–20in) tall and usually has whitish or purplish sepals and petals veined with purple and green, and a purple lip. It flowers in spring and early summer. This is one of those species that sometimes appears in lawns and anyone who is lucky enough to have a colony should be careful not to mow the grass until seed has been shed, usually at about the end of July or early in August.

Axil – the angle between a leaf and a stem

Bifoliate – with two leaves

Bract – a small leaf at the base of a flower stem or flower spike

Callus – a protruberance or growth, usually on the lip of an orchid

Clone – the asexually produced offspring of a single parent; they will be genetically identical

Column – in an orchid, the organ formed by the fusion of stamens, style and stigma

Cultivar – a particular form of a species or hybrid

Epiphyte – a plant which grows on another plant. but without obtaining nourishment from it

Genus (plural genera) – a natural group of closely related species

Grex – a group name for all plants derived from a cross between the same two species or hybrids

Intergeneric – between or among two or more genera

Intrageneric – within one genus

Keiki – a small plant arising from the stem, pseudobulb or inflorescence of a mature plant

Lip (labellum) – the unpaired petal of an orchid

Lithophyte – a plant which grows on a rock

Meristem – undifferentiated tissue, usually from a growing point, which is capable of developing into specialized tissue, used in mass propagation of orchids

Ovary – the part of a flower which contains the ovules and eventually becomes the fruit, containing seed

Pollinarium – the male reproductive part of an orchid flower, consisting of the pollinia from an anther with the associated parts, the viscidium and stipes

Pollinium (plural pollinia) – pollen grains cohering into a mass

Protocorm – A swollen, tuber-like structure that is the first stage of growth after an orchid seed germinates

Pseudobulb – a swollen, bulb–like structure at the base of a stem

Rhizome – a stem on or below the ground with roots growing down from it and flowering shoots up

Rupicolous – rock-dwelling

Species – a group of similar individuals, the basic unit of classification

Spur – a slender, usually hollow, extension of a flower, usually from the lip but in *Disa*, formed from the dorsal sepal

Stigma – the part of the column which receives pollen

Stipe or stipes (plural stipites) – a stalk joining the pollinium to the viscidium

Stolon – a running stem which forms roots

Synonym – botanically, another name for the same species which is now considered invalid

Terrestrial – growing in the ground

Unifoliate – with one leaf

Velamen – an absorbent layer of cells covering the roots of many orchids

Cover pictures: **Octopus Publishing Group Ltd.**/Mark Winwood

A-Z Botanical Collection 100, 98 Top, /Jiri Loun 99, 106 Bottom, /Terry Mead 17 Top, /Dan Sams 79, /Silvia Sroka 115, /Malkolm Warrington 118, 121, /Andy Williams 56 Top Left; **Adrian Bloom Horticultural Library**/Javier Delgado 16, 17 Bottom, 21, Professor Stefan Buczacki 35 left, 39; **Corbis UK Ltd**/Hal Horwitz 70 Top, 70 Bottom, 106 Top, /Kevin Schafer 67; **Eric Crichton** 59, 72 Top, 85; **DAC Photographics** 3, 36 left, 65, 78 right, 82, 109, 117; **Deni Bown** 69; **Garden Picture Library**/Mark Bolton 98 Bottom; **Garden & Wildlife Matters** 32, 36 right, 37 Bottom Right; **John Glover** 96 Top; **Octopus Publishing Group Ltd.** /John Sims 34, /Mark Winwood 1, 2, 4, 5, 10, 12 Bottom Right, 23, 24, 25, 26, 40, 41 Top, 41 Bottom, 42 Top, 42 Bottom, 43, 45, 48, 50, 54, 57, 58, 74, 84 Top, 92 Top, 92 Bottom, 94 Top, 97 Top, 104, 107, 112; **Harpur Garden Library**/Jerry Harpur 9, 56 Bottom Right, 72 Bottom, 80, 111, /Marcus Harpur 68 Top; **E.A.S. la Croix** 12 Top Left, 12 Top Right, 13 Top, 13 Bottom Right, 14, 62, 63, 76 Bottom, 77 Top, 83, 86 left, 86 right, 87, 89 Top, 89 Bottom, 93, 94 Bottom, 96 Bottom, 103, 120, 61, 91, 113; **Andrew Lawson** 119; **S & O Mathews** 55, 95 Top; **N.H.P.A.**/N.A.Callow 37 Top Right, /Kevin Schafer 101; **Oxford Scientific Films**/Raymond Blythe 64, /Deni Bown 77 Bottom, 84 Bottom, 102, /Peter Gould 73, /Geoff Kidd 60, 78 left, 81, 105, /R.L.Manuel 11, 20, 66, 71 Top, 76 Top, /Edward Parker 13 Bottom Left, /Kjell B Sandved 108; **Photos Horticultural** 27, 71 Bottom, 75, 68 Bottom, 90 Top, 90 Bottom; **Royal Horticultural Society** 53; **Science Photo Library**/Dr Jeremy Burgess 35 right, 37 left; **Harry Smith Collection** 88, 95 Bottom, 97 Bottom, 38.

AUTHOR'S ACKNOWLEDGEMENTS

I should like to thank my husband Eric, Joyce Stewart and Geoff Hands for help and advice in various ways.